DYAD
LEADERSHIP
and
CLINICAL
INTEGRATION

HAP

ACHE Management Series

DYAD
LEADERSHIP
and
CLINICAL
INTEGRATION

Driving Change,
Aligning Strategies

ALAN T. BELASEN

ACHE Management Series

Your board, staff, or clients may also benefit from this book's insight. For information on quantity discounts, contact the Health Administration Press Marketing Manager at (312) 424-9450.

This publication is intended to provide accurate and authoritative information in regard to the subject matter covered. It is sold, or otherwise provided, with the understanding that the publisher is not engaged in rendering professional services. If professional advice or other expert assistance is required, the services of a competent professional should be sought.

The statements and opinions contained in this book are strictly those of the author and do not represent the official positions of the American College of Healthcare Executives or the Foundation of the American College of Healthcare Executives.

23   22   21   20   19   5   4   3   2   1

Library of Congress Cataloging-in-Publication Data
Names: Belasen, Alan T., 1951- author.
Title: Dyad leadership and clinical integration : driving change, aligning
    strategies / Alan Belasen, PhD.
Description: Chicago, IL : Health Administration Press, 2019. | Series:
    HAP/ACHE management series.
Identifiers: LCCN 2019019783 (print) | LCCN 2019020228 (ebook) | ISBN
    9781640550919 (ebook) | ISBN 9781640550926 (xml) | ISBN 9781640550933
    (epub) | ISBN 9781640550940 (mobi) | ISBN 9781640550902 (pbk. : alk. paper)
Subjects: LCSH: Hospitals—Administration. | Leadership.
Classification: LCC RA971 (ebook) | LCC RA971 .B352 2019 (print) | DDC
    362.11068—dc23
LC record available at https://lccn.loc.gov/2019019783

The paper used in this publication meets the minimum requirements of American National Standard for Information Sciences—Permanence of Paper for Printed Library Materials, ANSI Z39.48-1984. ∞ ™

Acquisitions editor: Jennette McClain; Project manager: Theresa L. Rothschadl; Cover designer: Brad Norr; Layout: PerfecType

Found an error or a typo? We want to know! Please e-mail it to hapbooks@ache.org, mentioning the book's title and putting "Book Error" in the subject line.

For photocopying and copyright information, please contact Copyright Clearance Center at www.copyright.com or at (978) 750-8400.

Health Administration Press
A division of the Foundation of the American
    College of Healthcare Executives
300 S. Riverside Plaza, Suite 1900
Chicago, IL 60606–6698
(312) 424-2800

*To Susan Katz Belasen for her constant support,
sense of humor, and inspirational motivation.*

Contents

Foreword

OVER THE PAST decade and a half, I have served as a member of two hospital boards and reported to two other hospital or health system boards. I have witnessed the ever-increasing role of physicians in hospital governance and leadership.

In the environment I started in—academic medicine—the faculty, who were primarily physicians, have historically played a controlling role in administrative policies. There, the CEOs were not typically physicians, but because of the education mission of the hospital, many key members of the management team were. Academic health centers served as early models for the dyadic leadership that Alan Belasen's book espouses.

With an excellent grasp of contemporary healthcare issues and trends, Dr. Belasen addresses this emerging paradigm of physicians in hospital and health system leadership. He clearly articulates the need for top-level dyadic leadership as follows: "Administrators bring the business skills for providing cost-effective, sustainable delivery of care to broad populations. Physicians have the clinical expertise for ascertaining population health initiatives, caring for patients, and evaluating clinical outcomes." The focus of this book is optimizing success for hospital, health system, and accountable care organizations through partnered leadership. Specifically, Dr. Belasen describes the benefits of dyadic leadership for health innovation, population health initiatives, evidence-based approaches to medicine, effective team building, efficiency, and costs. The identification and development of physician leaders are themes woven throughout the book.

Later in my career, I joined a community hospital board. At that time, the concept of dyadic leadership was just emerging in community hospitals and was viewed as essential in the "patient-centeredness" mandates of the board and external agencies. It was interesting for me to observe, in a nonacademic environment, the imperative to engage physicians in hospital management decisions. I witnessed firsthand the angst that physician involvement in management created. These stresses are still apparent today, as physician members of governing boards are often criticized for having self-serving motives in their decision-making and advocacy efforts. Indeed, there is much written and said about inappropriate and appropriate physician involvement in hospital boards (e.g., the writings of James E. Orlikoff, president of Orlikoff & Associates, Inc., and a member of the American Hospital Association Speakers Bureau).

Regardless of the struggle to find the right paradigm of physician involvement, fostering such involvement is worth the effort. The healthcare field has widely recognized that physician participation at the very top of healthcare organizations enhances the quality of care (e.g., the American Association for Physician Leadership patient-centered care initiative, which champions physician leadership as essential).

The concepts articulated in Belasen's *Dyad Leadership and Clinical Integration* are consistent with other emerging imperatives in medicine—for example, those of interprofessional education and team-based medicine. In the former, medical students and students in healthcare management, nursing, public health, dentistry, social work, pharmacy, and allied health disciplines learn together in teams. In the latter, each member of the multidisciplinary team must appreciate knowledge and skills that other members bring to the table. Both require a flattening of the hierarchical approach to medicine, with a sole doctor on the top.

In parallel with the move away from the patriarchy of the physician leader in medicine, Dr. Belasen suggests a specific structure that departs from the historic structure of an administratively trained CEO (typically with a master's degree in business administration or health administration) who is alone at the helm of the hospital or health system. The newly proposed structure is a dyad of an administrator and a physician to lead such organizations jointly.

Dr. Belasen illustrates how in this post–Affordable Care Act, post–American Health Care Act era, and with its environment defined by value-based purchasing, this approach is essential.

Applying a paradigm he is well known for—the competing values framework—Dr. Belasen guides potential and newly formed dyads toward optimal functioning, full communication, and the ability to discern training gaps. His exhibits, articulating the major domains of operation in health systems—cross-referenced with the responsibilities of the administrative leader, the physician leader, and the dyad's shared responsibilities—are especially helpful, as is the application of the balanced scorecard to health system administration. He also provides an assessment tool for established dyads, in which either the individual skills (e.g., emotional intelligence, personality traits, communication styles) or the interpersonal interactions within the dyad may be functioning at a subpar level. Dr. Belasen's easy-to-generate, usable graphic displays of assessment results enable ready detection of deficiencies. Remedies for many deficiencies are suggested.

Using actual examples, Dr. Belasen illustrates how the assessment tools have been used to increase team effectiveness. Other examples of organizations that have successfully engaged dyadic leadership are given. Thus, no matter where an individual or organization may be on the road toward a goal of dyadic leadership, *Dyad Leadership and Clinical Integration* can assist in the journey.

Dr. Laura Schweitzer
President Emeritus, Union Graduate College
Vice President for Health Sciences at the University at Albany, State University of New York

Acknowledgments

I AM GRATEFUL and indebted to the colleagues, clinicians, and experts who contributed valuable ideas and suggestions to earlier drafts. I would like to acknowledge the insights and feedback of Dr. Richard Boehler, former president and CEO of St. Joseph Hospital, Nashua, NH, who provided me with critical insights that deepened my understanding of today's complex healthcare environments and the leadership challenges associated with clinical and operational alignment.

I benefited from the advice and wisdom of many colleagues from numerous networks and associations, including the Association of University Programs in Health Administration, the American College of Healthcare Executives, and the Academy of Management. Special thanks go to Dr. Laura Schweitzer, president emeritus of Union Graduate College and vice president for health sciences at the University at Albany, State University of New York (SUNY), who wrote the foreword to the book. Laura involved me in executive education and leadership development programs and influenced my thinking about entrepreneurial leadership.

Abigail Belasen, MD, resident in internal medicine at Mount Sinai Health System, offered useful feedback and constructive criticism of many ideas relating to the importance of interfunctional collaboration, improving the quality of the patient experience, and physician–patient communication.

Dr. John Huppertz, chair of the healthcare management master's program at the David D. Reh School of Business of Clarkson University, and Dr. Martin A. Strosberg, professor in the bioethics program of Clarkson University and the Ihcan School of Medicine at Mount Sinai, offered critical thoughts and ideas that shaped the direction of *Dyad Leadership and Clinical Integration*. My students in the master's of business administration in healthcare program at SUNY Empire State College and in the School of Business at Clarkson University provided me with the opportunity to answer questions and to think more deeply about the attributes of effective leadership in complex healthcare environments.

The constructive feedback that I received from anonymous reviewers through Health Administration Press (HAP) and the focused suggestions from HAP's editorial review board on earlier drafts of the proposed book helped shape the scope and directions of *Dyad Leadership*. Many thanks to my HAP acquisitions editor, Jennette McClain, whose enthusiastic endorsement of my original idea and constant support along the way facilitated the production of this book from start to finish. Special thanks go to Theresa Rothschadl, editor, HAP, who was instrumental in not only making sure that the manuscript follows the publisher's editorial guidelines but also for offering critical review that facilitated the format and improved the clarity and flow of ideas, visuals, and narratives. Thanks to Andrew Baumann, editorial production manager, for setting up the logistical framework and coordinating the various phases of the book production.

My wife, Susan, provided me with social and emotional support, as well as a sounding board for many of the ideas in this book. Sharing or discussing its concepts with my five As was especially inspiring and thought-provoking: Ari, an accomplished scholar and professor of economics; Amy, an author and a marketing consultant; Anat, who very soon will be receiving her PhD in ecology and evolutionary biology from the University of Michigan, Ann Arbor, and has been awarded a David H. Smith postdoctoral Conservation Research fellowship, which she will carry out in collaboration with Cornell University; Amanda, with a master's degree in communication; and Abigail, a physician with Mount Sinai. I am deeply indebted to all of you.

CHAPTER 1

Aims and Scope

INTRODUCTION

In the upheaval of today's healthcare system, with its push toward clinical integration, what leadership model will produce stability, even progress? *Dyad Leadership and Clinical Integration* establishes that developing and sustaining dyad leadership is compatible with the growing complexity of the healthcare environment and its many major changes. In fact, the interdisciplinary structure of the dyad aligns well with the drive toward clinical integration.

As you read, you will learn how to use assessment tools to examine the efficacy of the dyad structure and improve hospital management. Further, you will be able to evaluate how well the partners in the dyad complement each other and suggest ways to improve their combined strengths and abilities.

Assessment instruments are designed to help increase self-awareness of one's strengths, weaknesses, thinking patterns, and motivations. Stakeholders (e.g., board members) can use these instruments to identify potential gaps in the skills and competencies of leaders at all levels and make important decisions about investments in leadership development programs. As such, the assessment instruments provided in this book will allow you to contextualize leadership roles and competencies and align them with the goals and strategies of your healthcare system. The framework helps dyads navigate the hazards of competing values and contradictory interests successfully, making better, more informed decisions. Its central feature is the relationship among strategy, structure, and leadership roles.

PURPOSE OF THE BOOK

This book focuses primarily on complementary forms of leadership and on effective collaboration among physicians, managers, and trustees. We will examine the evolving role of executive dyads in navigating the transition toward value-based systems, laying out a fresh set of collaborative methods that increase leadership effectiveness and accountability. The book highlights the importance of combining clinical competence with administrative skills, mastering leadership and communication competencies, relentlessly pushing to improve the patient experience, and initiating measures to reduce risk and increase safety and reliability.

With leaders drawn solely from management programs, healthcare organizations run the risk of lopsided leadership. Executives who climb the corporate ladder without a deep understanding of the complexity of clinical environments—and of patient flow and cycle time—often fail to recognize how physicians think, decide, and act. Moreover, unlike the usual supervisory structure of management teams in other sectors, which operate through hierarchical reporting, clinical leaders rely on a collegial orientation. In contrast to administrators, clinical leaders focus on patient service. Executives with a management background are sometimes at a loss to understand, let alone improve, the functioning of their own institutions.

What happens when executives and clinical staff work as partners, however? The combination of clinical competence and administrative skills allows the dyad, especially at the executive level, to inform data-driven innovation, pursue wise technology upgrades, and master competitive pressures. This synergy leads to smarter choices in electronic health record implementation, resource allocation, and focused capital investments.

ALIGNMENT OF WORK WITH STRATEGY

An expanded role for physicians in hospital leadership is paramount to the success of clinical integration—a shared vision of a value-based culture in a hospital or healthcare network. However, the question of *how* to involve physicians is difficult to approach; value and integration will likely require structural ambidexterity and leadership skills for managing paradoxes.

In keeping with the maxim "structure follows strategy," health systems benefit when they are configured to be compatible with their strategy—from the creation of divisions and departments to the designation of reporting relationships. In addition, centering the organization's strategic objectives helps achieve the mission and goals of the integrated health system, one in which leadership development programs and skill-building initiatives are aligned with strategic objectives. For example, the strategy of providing health services across the continuum of care through partnerships and alliances at the macro level is supported with interprofessional teamwork at the micro level.

By aligning roles and skills with business objectives, top executives can ensure that the investments they make in leadership development and succession planning are linked with the strategic direction of the organization. Alignment gives organizational members a sense of shared purpose and an understanding of organizational goals and mission. They develop a better sense of ownership, become more committed and accountable, and work collaboratively to achieve aims. Energy and inspiration run high, and both individual and team effectiveness increase.

TRANSFORMATIONS IN THE HEALTHCARE FIELD

Since the advent of the Affordable Care Act (ACA), hospitals have faced enormous pressure to transition from the acute care model. They now work to provide cost-effective health services organizations with a full range of offerings. Executives work hard to align incentives for providers with quality goals. They seek to integrate care services and delivery, ranging from inpatient and ancillary services (e.g., audiology, clinical lab services) to home health, occupational and physical therapy, pharmacies, and nursing homes.

Simultaneously, a significant convergence across healthcare fields is occurring, blurring the lines between payers and providers. Integration takes place clinically or financially, horizontally or vertically. With the rising demand for improved facilities, superior equipment, and new medical technology, and as hospitals look to scale up and improve, mergers are becoming a key growth strategy.

The consolidation of hospitals into integrated healthcare systems, with initiatives ranging from loose affiliations and nonequity agreements to formal partnerships and complete mergers, requires new models of executive leadership. In subsequent chapters, I will demonstrate how dyad leadership aligns well with the strategic initiatives of healthcare systems.

SIZE MATTERS

In the consumer-driven marketplace, achieving economies of scale is a key competitive strategy for large healthcare organizations. Consolidation allows the parties to control costs by reducing or eliminating redundancy, making it possible to reap the benefits of cost advantage and increased efficiencies. Economies of scale are also critical for sustaining the big data analytics that hold considerable promise for effectively managing care delivery.

Recently, a wave of mergers, acquisitions, and partnerships has begun to alter the structure of healthcare systems. In 1975, there were 7,156 hospitals in the United States (National Center for Health Statistics 2017). As exhibit 1.1 shows, however, by 2010 (pre-ACA), the total number of hospitals had dropped by about 1,400. Since then, it has continued to decrease, primarily as a result of closing or consolidation. By 2015, the number of hospitals stood at 5,564,

Exhibit 1.1: Number of US Hospitals

	1975	1980	1990	2000	2005	2010	2012	2013	2014	2015
All hospitals	7,156	6,965	6,649	5,810	5,756	5,754	5,723	5,686	5,627	5,564
Federal	382	359	337	245	226	213	211	213	213	212
Nonfederal	6,774	6,606	6,312	5,565	5,530	5,541	5,512	5,473	5,414	5,352
Community	5,875	5,830	5,384	4,915	4,936	4,985	4,999	4,974	4,926	4,862
Nonprofit	3,339	3,322	3,191	3,003	2,958	2,904	2,894	2,904	2,870	2,845
For profit	775	730	749	749	868	1,013	1,068	1,060	1,053	1,034
State or local government	1,761	1,778	1,444	1,163	1,110	1,068	1,037	1,010	1,003	983

Source: National Center for Health Statistics (2017).

with the majority registered as nongovernment, not-for-profit community hospitals (2,845) and for-profit institutions (1,034), followed by state or local government hospitals (983) (American Hospital Association 2017).

Across the country, megasystems that control an increasing share of the market are changing their business models, consolidating services in regional hubs and creating a competitive edge. Many facilities have become, in effect, outpatient clinics (Ross 2018). Large and financially stable multihospital systems have been racing to form megasystems, in an attempt get ahead of the ACA mandate to improve quality and increase efficiency through coordinated care across the entire care continuum.

Alongside their growth in size and market share, hospital or health system ownership of physician practices grew also by 86 percent from 2012 to 2015. According to Physicians Advocacy Institute (2016) research, 67,000 physician practices nationwide were hospital-owned in 2015, with 38 percent of physicians employed by health systems.

By the end of 2017, a new wave of unprecedented mergers among the largest Catholic-owned hospital systems in the nation took place, with the aim of further strengthening their brands and health services. Combined, the Dignity Health and Catholic Health integrated system reportedly includes 700 care sites, as well as 139 hospitals staffed by 159,000 employees, including more than 25,000 physicians and other advanced-practice clinicians (Dignity Health 2017). Ascension and Providence St. Joseph Health also plan to create a nonprofit health system giant with nearly 200 hospitals across 27 states (Evans and Mathews 2017). Other Catholic systems have already bought hospitals from for-profit chains.

The pace of consolidation in healthcare has led many independent hospitals to consider joining or affiliating with other organizations. While some hospitals have formed partnerships and collaborations to improve clinical and financial outcomes, others have consolidated long-term and post-acute services and moved discharge planning and transition management across the spectrum of care under common leadership.

Economies of scale, however, have negative side effects or mitigating factors, called diseconomies of scale. While multihospital networks and merged health systems enjoy increased bargaining power with payers, oversized organizations create economic disadvantages as a result of their new complexity. This complexity also yields additional cost, which outweighs the savings gained from greater scale.

With more hospitals, physician networks, and health systems consolidating under common leadership, achieving a sustainable clinical and operational alignment across specialties and networks is becoming increasingly challenging, both functionally and organizationally.

CHANGES IN LEADERSHIP ROLES

With the expansion of the corporate office in megasystems, local healthcare CEOs experience increased centralization and decreased autonomy. Local boards are becoming advisory in nature. Local cultures are becoming more corporatized, and the focus of the local CEO is changing from strategic or visionary planning to operational duties. "True" CEOs are far fewer in number. Even the titles are changing—the healthcare sector is now led by presidents, senior vice presidents, and chief administrative officers. One consequence of these changes is a significant increase in CEO turnover rates, which exceeded 20 percent for the first time in 2013 and averaged more than 17 percent over 2012–2017 (American College of Healthcare Executives 2017).

In New York State, the department of health continues to require a local board for each hospital that is generally subservient to a parent board, which in turn has certain reserve power over the local boards. Though the extent to which a local CEO reports to a governing board or corporate officers often reflects her hospital's structure and affiliation, she often reports to a local board and a parent (i.e., integrated system) CEO. You can imagine the complexity of matrix relationships that result.

In virtually every state, and across state lines, the rate of hospital transactions and partnerships is accelerating with direct effects on the local CEO. Each facility, though, continues to need an "officer in charge" or, possibly, a dyad to run the local operations effectively.

SYNERGY AS STRATEGY

With the increase in size and complexity of health systems, it becomes more challenging for a single leader to possess the skills, knowledge, or perspectives necessary for optimal decisions. A supervisory structure with clear lines of authority, driven primarily by nonclinical administrators, is less suited to today's challenges.

Dyads, which pair an administrator with a physician partner, create a powerful synergy that reinforces the new business model. A 2014 survey conducted by the Advisory Board (Trandel 2015) showed that dyad leaders operate in multiple locations within health systems, including the C-suite (e.g., chief medical officer, chief quality officer), divisions of care providers (e.g., regional primary care network, health centers), and even service lines (e.g., cardiovascular, orthopedics, cancer care). The dyad is congruent with the growth strategy of integrated health systems. The coleaders collaborate to achieve shared goals in their respective positions.

Dyads allow leaders to turn their differences into advantages, cultivating the joint thinking that leads to optimal decisions. Administrators bring the business skills vital to cost-effective, sustainable delivery of care to broad populations. Physicians have the clinical expertise for selecting population health initiatives, caring for patients, and evaluating clinical outcomes. The effective functioning of dyads requires a culture of partnership between administrators and physicians, with a dual focus on flexibility and control, transformational and transactional roles, open communication, and consistency in operations.

Not every physician or executive is well suited for coleadership. According to the Physician Leadership Forum (2014), four characteristics are vital for aspiring physician leaders:

1. The complexity of healthcare organizations requires strong leaders from within the field. Physicians with substantial knowledge of issues such as access, quality, safety improvement, and patient care are more suited to lead health systems than physicians who are not interested in these topics.
2. Physicians with the capacity to embrace a culture of interprofessional collaboration are better positioned to succeed.
3. Physicians who place a high priority on supplementing their functional knowledge and academic skills with leadership development and management skills are prepared for successful leadership.
4. Physicians transitioning into leadership roles must recognize the need for additional skills as they pursue leadership success.

FOCUS

Throughout, *Dyad Leadership and Clinical Integration* maps the dyadic leadership capabilities that extend beyond the traditional roles of hospital executives. The book also offers advice from hospital leaders and other experts about how to achieve an optimal alignment between the dyad management structure and the hospital's strategic priorities. After reading this book, you should be motivated to change your approach to leading and managing healthcare systems. You will also be inspired to pursue a leadership education and development path to achieve your career advancement goal.

Important questions about the effectiveness of the dyad, covered in this book, include the following:

- What is the context (institutional, organizational, operational) for dyad leadership in a health system?
- How are physicians and administrators paired? How do we optimize the complementary roles and strengths of the partners in a way that makes the dyad more relevant and accountable to organizational goals and needs?
- How can partners sustain trust, mutual respect, and common understanding over time?
- How do we ensure the existence of leadership capacity among physicians with the potential to lead their organizations?

KEY TAKEAWAYS

- Achieving a sustainable clinical and operational alignment across the continuum of care is becoming increasingly complex.
- Cooperative decision-making and interprofessional teamwork are necessary for dealing with complexity.

- New positions have been added to C-suites, roles and responsibilities are evolving, and leadership titles are being redefined.
- The interdisciplinary structure of dyad leadership aligns well with contemporary healthcare goals.
- A successful dyad is built on trust, mutual respect, and complementary skill.
- The combined strength of dyad leadership generates influence and synergy greater than the sum of their parts.
- Using assessment instruments facilitates understanding across administrative levels and functional lines.
- The assessment framework clarifies the relationships among strategy, structure, and leadership roles.
- Aligning roles and skills with healthcare goals and strategies helps to link leadership development to the strategic direction of the health system.
- Economies of scale improve integration of care and reduce duplication; however, diseconomies must be monitored and managed carefully.

REFERENCES

American College of Healthcare Executives. 2017. "Hospital CEO Turnover Rate Remains Steady." Published June 14. www.ache.org/learning-center/research/about-ceos/hospital-ceo-turnover/hospital-ceo-turnover-rate-2017.

American Hospital Association. 2017. "Fast Facts on US Hospitals 2017." Published January. www.aha.org/statistics/fast-facts-us-hospitals-2017.

Dignity Health. 2017. "Dignity Health and Catholic Health Initiatives to Combine to Form New Catholic Health System Focused on Creating Healthier Communities." Published December 7.

www.dignityhealth.org/about-us/press-center/press-releases/
dignity-health-and-catholic-health-initiatives-announcement.

Evans, M., and A. W. Mathews. 2017. "Hospital Giants in Talks
to Merge to Create Nation's Largest Operator." *Wall Street
Journal*. Published December 10. www.wsj.com/articles/
hospital-giants-in-talks-to-merge-to-create-nations-largest
-operator-1512921420.

National Center for Health Statistics. 2017. *Health, United States,
2016: With Chartbook on Long-Term Trends in Health*. Centers
for Disease Control and Prevention, US Department of Health
and Human Services. Published May. www.cdc.gov/nchs/data/
hus/hus16.pdf.

Physicians Advocacy Institute. 2016. "Physician Practice Acquisi-
tion Study: National and Regional Employment Changes."
Published September. www.physiciansadvocacyinstitute.org/
Portals/0/assets/docs/PAI-Physician-Employment-Study.pdf.

Physician Leadership Forum. 2014. *Physician Leadership Education*.
American Hospital Association. Accessed December 17, 2018.
www.ahaphysicianforum.org/files/pdf/LeadershipEducation
.pdf.

Ross, C. 2018. "Paying More and Getting Less: As Hospital Chains
Grow, Local Services Shrink." *STAT*. Published January 24.
www.statnews.com/2018/01/24/hospital-chains-services
-consolidation/.

Trandel, E. 2015. "Advocating for Dyad Leadership at Your Organization? Use Our Slides." Advisory Board. Published March
26. www.advisory.com/research/physician-executive-council/
prescription-for-change/2015/03/dyad-leadership.

Dyad Leadership: An Integrated Approach

Exhibit 1: Dyad Leadership in Transforming Healthcare Systems

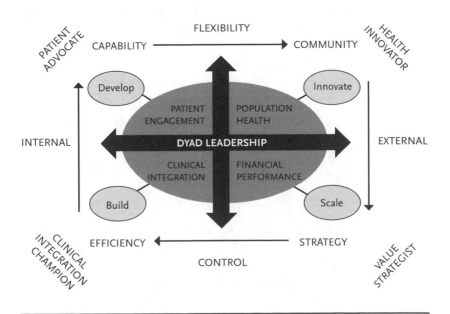

Part I explores a framework, developed specifically for this book, for contextualizing the roles and responsibilities of dyad leaders.

The framework is rooted in organizational effectiveness criteria; therefore, it serves to link leadership roles with organizational goals. Using the ideas explored in this book, dyad leaders can view their health system holistically.

The framework provides a lens for physicians and administrators through which to group and differentiate roles and competencies for optimal outcomes. This tool helps to align complementary leadership roles and competencies with the guiding strategy of the organization. Chapter 2 examines ambidexterity and the dyad management structure as concepts and systems compatible with complex healthcare environments. Chapter 3 presents the integrated framework that serves as an organizing schema for the book. The framework is also used as a road map for contextualizing the dyad leadership roles and domains of operations. Moreover, it provides important anchors for the assessment instruments that were developed specifically for this book. Chapter 4 presents a method for diagnosing and analyzing dyad roles, with examples and interpretations.

Complexity and Ambidexterity

INTRODUCTION

The supervisory structure of traditional hospitals—a single authority line, typically led by nonclinical administrators—is ill suited to the complexity of multihospital settings. In contrast, the dyad—which pairs an administrator with a physician partner—aligns well with the complex structure of integrated health systems. This interdisciplinary structure is synergistic, and it contributes effectively to patient care; engagement; and joint accountability by team members, patients, and families.

Chapter 2 argues that an ambidextrous structure can anchor dyad leadership. *Ambidextrous management* focuses on a dual logic. The first logic is humanistic or collaborative, used to develop ideas and initiate innovation. The second logic is managerial or rationalistic, concerned with the efficient use of resources to implement innovation. This dual focus matches the conditions for a successful dyad, which pairs clinical and administrative champions to facilitate the transformation to value-based care and population health.

BUNDLED PAYMENTS FIT THE INTERDISCIPLINARY STRUCTURE

The dyad management structure is congruent with complex healthcare environments and with the shift to cost-effective health service programs across the continuum of care. The move away from fee-for-service payment can be facilitated with collaborative forms of management that include physicians.

Common funding models, such as fee-for-service, are fragmented. Because they focus on individual episodes of care, they are less compatible with coordinated or collaborative delivery. Payments tend to reward the quantity of services offered by providers rather than the quality of care provided.

Bundled payments, which link reimbursement for the multiple services beneficiaries have received during an episode of care, enable more efficient care delivery by providing incentives for a better patient experience and higher levels of productivity using the same resources. When the Centers for Medicare & Medicaid Services began reducing Medicare payments for hospitals with excess readmissions through the Inpatient Prospective Payment System, hospitals used various means to discourage patients from making a U-turn after discharge. However, a recent study published in *JAMA: The Journal of the American Medical Association* found that as hospitals initiated a reduction in readmissions for heart failure patients, mortality rates also began to increase (Gupta et al. 2017). Bundled payments align incentives for providers (i.e., hospitals, post-acute care providers, physicians, other practitioners), allowing them to work closely together across specialties and settings.

Bundled payments also fit the interdisciplinary structure of the dyad management model, which aligns well with the cooperative decision-making and interprofessional collaboration necessary for managing the complexity of healthcare organizations.

INTEGRATION AND TRUST

With the intensity of consolidation in healthcare, the number of stand-alone hospitals is diminishing quickly. Even critical access hospitals have been affected by this change. This trend is magnified by the formation of alliances and partnerships, as well as local and

The Value of Physician Leadership

Health care organizations need the distinctive perspective of physicians among their leadership. Because of increased constraints on revenue and heightened review by payers, health system leaders of today are now more often in the position of making administrative decisions that ultimately affect clinical care. . . .

ACPE [The American College of Physician Executives] includes physician leadership as one of its nine essential elements required to provide optimal patient-centered care. . . . To succeed, health care must be: quality-centered, safe, streamlined, measured, evidence-based, value-driven, innovative, fair and equitable, and physician-led.

—Peter Angood and Susan Birk (2014)

regional nonequity network relationships of health systems, which work together more closely toward coordinated and improved care.

For example, accountable care organizations (ACOs) are on the rise, though their individual solutions to the problem of alliance vary widely. They typically do not use an ownership model or a merger. Instead, ACOs often opt for a partnership model, whereby members cooperate under an ACO participation agreement while retaining their independence. Some healthcare systems operate as relatively loose confederations of independent hospitals. Others have gone further by instituting explicit policies and standards that all members follow. Some are vertically integrated structures comprising multiple complementary organizations.

Regardless of their methods of cooperation, hospitals throughout the United States have had to adjust to functioning on an interconnected basis. Being part of a bigger organization allows them economies of scale in various areas, including staff sharing and joint purchasing. However, with greater integration, sustaining alignment is increasingly complex and challenging. In the process, concerns about trust, communication, and leadership effectiveness have been mounting.

COMMUNICATION AND TRUST

When healthcare workers were asked by Willis Towers Watson how accessible, open, and honest their leaders' communication was, employees have increasingly graded executives down. Opinions started to decline in favorability in 2012–2013 and leveled off, with no improvement, by the close of 2015. This downward progress suggests that, as pressures on the business model linked to healthcare reform started to build, employees began to listen for more information on plans and performance. In the process, they became more critical of leaders' ability to reach workers and the veracity of the messages heard from the top ranks. It appears as if, broadly speaking, leaders have missed an opportunity to engage employees in the changes needed to adjust to the new dynamics in the healthcare sector (Kulesa 2016).

Dyad leaders create synergistic work environments that promote mutual trust and joint accountability. Instituting a dyad management structure embeds physician leaders in the supervisory structure and creates opportunities for dealing with complexity through collaboration. By communicating vision and strategy, dyad leaders encourage team members to share a high level of commitment and use teamwork to achieve broader, emerging goals.

COMPLEXITY AND AMBIDEXTERITY

In the vocabulary of management scholarship (Kannampallil et. al. 2011), entities that evolve in a network of interdependent

Healthcare System Complexities

In his presentation [for the Institute of Medicine,] William W. Stead, chief information officer of Vanderbilt University Medical Center, described the current healthcare environment as characterized by competition, misaligned incentives, and inherent distrust among stakeholders. Throughout healthcare, Stead sees competing cultures at loggerheads—as exemplified by the tensions among consumers who want high service and low out-of-pocket costs, payers who want to select risk and limit cost, and purchasers who want more value at the lowest cost. Looking to a future that will be defined by individualized medicine, Stead suggested that tomorrow's opportunities might not be fully realized without fundamental changes in the culture. Education for health professionals is only one area that needs reform. Another requirement will be to move from the business of managing episodes of care to the business of caring for patients and populations. He added that similar fundamental reforms will need to be incorporated into the business models of virtually every healthcare stakeholder—in payment mechanisms, and, notably, in the role of the individuals in managing their own care.

—Institute of Medicine and National Academy of Engineering (2011)

organizations are characterized as *complex adaptive systems* (CAS). To accomplish goals, these systems draw on nonlinear (i.e., unpredictable) processes, emergent goals, and coevolution (i.e., a series of reciprocally induced changes between interacting systems) with all other linked systems. CAS display high levels of member engagement, coevolution, balanced exploration and exploitation, disruptive innovation, and reintegration and disintegration of structures and processes. (*Exploitation* is behaviors and activities that optimize performance in current tasks, and *exploration* is behaviors and activities leading to disengagement from current tasks in pursuit of new alternatives.) Typically, a decision or action by one part in the system affects interrelated parts, but not necessarily in any uniform manner. The success of CAS depends on striking a balance between exploiting existing resources (or core competencies) and exploring new resources and capabilities.

Complex adaptive systems rely on dynamics of punctuated equilibrium (switching between long-term stability and rapid change) to transform and self-organize into structures more compatible for handling disruptive innovation. In healthcare fields, this may trigger health systems with ambidextrous governance and hybrid technologies and processes that function in both high- and low-end markets. Ambidexterity separates the daily operations and optimization of current capabilities from those focused on innovative thinking and transforming the way care is delivered. The employment of hybrid operating rooms, for example, increases utilization, enhances patient safety, reduces overall cost, and increases clinical staff satisfaction (*Becker's Hospital Review* 2011). Ambidexterity requires the willingness of senior managers to commit resources to exploratory projects and the establishment of separate structural units for exploitation and exploration (O'Reilly and Tushman 2004). The challenge of transforming health systems is to configure and reconfigure organizational resources to capture existing as well as new opportunities by relying on management actions that facilitate the simultaneous pursuit of exploitation and exploration. This book argues that the dyad leadership structure allows health systems to develop greater ambidexterity as they search for better ways to balance practices supporting optimal exploitation of existing resources and exploring new ways to accomplish strategic objectives.

Reframing the Challenges to Integrated Care: A Complex-Adaptive Systems Perspective

Our findings indicate that integration is challenged by system complexity, weak ties and poor alignment among professionals and organizations, a lack of funding incentives to support collaborative work, and a bureaucratic environment based on a command and control approach to management. Using a CAS framework, we identified several characteristics of CAS in our data, including diverse, interdependent and semi-autonomous actors; embedded co-evolutionary systems; emergent behaviors and non-linearity; and self-organizing capacity. . . .

One possible explanation for the lack of systems change towards integration is that we have failed to treat the healthcare system as complex-adaptive. The data suggest that future integration initiatives must be anchored in a CAS perspective, and focus on building the system's capacity to self-organize. We conclude that integrating care requires policies and management practices that promote system awareness, relationship-building and information-sharing, and that recognize change as an evolving learning process rather than a series of programmatic steps.

—Peter Tsasis, Jenna M. Evans, and Susan Owen (2012)

The next chapter covers the main tenets of the integrated approach. As you will see, the dimensions and quadrants of the framework match the complexity of the healthcare environment.

KEY TAKEAWAYS

- Dyad leaders use their combined strengths to understand, analyze, and deal with complex healthcare challenges.
- Dyad leaders need to have a shared strategy, pursuing both exploitation and exploration proactively.
- Hospitals' strategic orientation toward alliances and partnerships can be explained by the framework of ambidexterity and exploration versus exploitation.

Performance Improvement in Hospitals: Leveraging on Knowledge Asset Dynamics Through the Introduction of an Electronic Medical Record

A first element emerging from all the three cases is that—focusing on producing, finding, analyzing and sharing information through digital media—EMR [electronic medical records] manifests its ambidextrous potential in triggering and enabling augmented capabilities in knowledge exploration and knowledge exploitation by increasing the coordination among hospital processes. The CEO of one of the hospitals stated: "I've always thought of ICT as a lever to cut costs. As a matter of fact, there are tremendous benefits in terms of quality improvement as well: once you connect the different departments, you discover new and better ways to provide healthcare services and have an impact on patients' outcome."

—Luca Gastaldi et al. (2012)

- Opportunities for exploitation include current business structures, management practices and processes, solutions to current performance issues, established practices, and risk-averse behaviors.
- Organizations can explore transformational leadership, innovative thinking, inquiry, behavioral flexibility, experimentation, and risk-taking.
- Dyads use combined strengths to do the following:
  - Develop new delivery models and cater to community needs
  - Pursue partnerships to strengthen finance and sustain market share
  - Reduce costs by improving compliance and operating efficiencies
  - Improve physician and patient engagement
- To sustain the dyad approach, leaders should focus on developing physician leadership and on succession planning that identifies, cultivates, and selects physician coleaders.
- To ensure successful outcomes, champion leadership development programs and skill-building opportunities that align organizational needs with systemwide leadership capability.
- The integrated approach can help to group and differentiate the unique roles and competencies of dyad leaders within the context of organizational needs and goals.

REFERENCES

Angood, P., and S. Birk. 2014. "The Value of Physician Leadership." *Physician Executive* 40 (3): 6–20.

Becker's Hospital Review. 2011. "4 Benefits of a Hybrid Operating Room." Published June 28. www.beckershospitalreview.com/or-efficiencies/4-benefits-of-a-hybrid-operating-room.html.

Gastaldi, L., E. Lettieri, M. Mariano Corso, and C. Masella. 2012. "Performance Improvement in Hospitals: Leveraging on Knowledge Asset Dynamics Through the Introduction of an Electronic Medical Record." *Measuring Business Excellence* 16 (4): 14–30.

Gupta A., L. A. Allen, D. L. Bhatt, M. Cox, A. D. DeVore, P. A. Heidenreich, A. F. Hernandez, E. D. Peterson, R. A. Matsouaka, C. W. Yancy, and G. C. Fonarow. 2017. "Association of the Hospital Readmissions Reduction Program Implementation with Readmission and Mortality Outcomes in Heart Failure." *JAMA Cardiology* 3 (1): 44–53.

Institute of Medicine and National Academy of Engineering. 2011. *Engineering a Learning Healthcare System: A Look at the Future.* Washington, DC: National Academies Press. https://doi.org/10.17226/12213.

Kannampallil, T. G., G. F. Schauer, T. Cohen, and V. Patel. 2011. "Considering Complexity in Healthcare Systems." *Journal of Biomedical Informatics* 44 (6): 943–47.

Kulesa, P. 2016. "Leadership in Crisis: Healthcare Workers Grow More Critical of Top Management Post-reform." *Becker's Hospital Review*. Published June 23. www.beckershospitalreview .com/hospital-management-administration/leadership-in-crisis -healthcare-workers-grow-more-critical-of-top-management -post-reform.html.

O'Reilly, C. A., and M. L. Tushman. 2004. "The Ambidextrous Organization." *Harvard Business Review* 82 (4): 74–81.

Tsasis, P., J. Evans, and S. Owen. 2012. "Reframing the Challenges to Integrated Care: A Complex-Adaptive Systems Perspective." *International Journal of Integrated Care* 12 (5): e190.

CHAPTER 3

An Integrated Approach

INTRODUCTION

This chapter introduces a version of a competing values framework (exhibits 3.1, 3.2). The competing values framework is a model used to study organizational effectiveness, mapping values according to two intersecting axes: from flexibility to control and from internal to external. Our modified framework is designed specifically to consider healthcare organizational performance and to align leadership roles with important domains of operations: innovation, scale, building, and development.

The competing values framework generally encourages leaders to view tasks and responsibilities from a unified "both/and" perspective, rather than a binary "either/or" perspective. The framework transcends apparent paradoxes to identify win–win solutions (Cameron and Quinn 2006).

The framework discussed in this book can be used as a diagnostic tool or a communication assessment tool, and it can be used to assist in leadership development. When employed to assess the effectiveness of leadership roles or communication styles, it helps facilitate understanding of information, meaning, roles, and behaviors used by partners in the dyad or by executives and clinical leaders who interact in decision situations. Chapter 4 illustrates these assessments.

Exhibit 3.1: Competing Values Framework: Healthcare Leadership

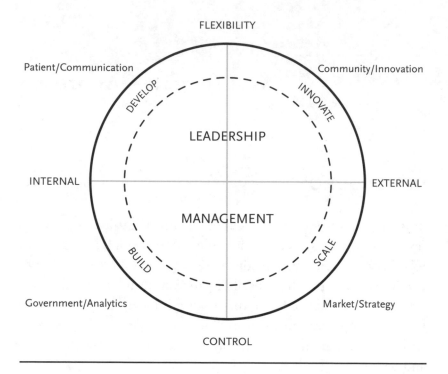

Dyad leaders can also use the framework for articulating message orientations (how they select the right approach to communicating tasks and goals) and the impact of messages on stakeholders' perceptions (Belasen 2008). Chapter 24 discusses these techniques in more depth. As a leadership development tool, the framework helps to identify leaders' strengths and weaknesses and to provide insights about the training required to close potential leadership gaps (Belasen, Eisenberg, and Huppertz 2015). Chapters 25 and 26 discuss this use in detail in the context of competency development.

Subsequent parts of the book examine how executives can use this framework for self-assessment and continuous improvement.

In this chapter, however, we take a closer look at the framework: its axes, terminology, and relevance to dyad leadership.

MANAGEMENT AND LEADERSHIP

Before we discuss the use of the competing values framework in healthcare, we should first consider the basic differences between leadership and management. There is no question that both leadership and management are demanding, challenging, and vital to the successful operation of healthcare organizations. However, the two have different orientations.

Management is centered on performance, seeking to maintain stability, predictability, and order. Managers are responsible for attaining organizational goals as rationally as possible through planning, organizing, and controlling organizational resources. They use centralized authority to direct employees.

Leadership, in contrast, is centered on the members of the organization. Hierarchical relations do not bind leaders. While managers use administrative power (e.g., reward, punishment) to attain goals, leadership creates change in a culture of integrity, helping the organization thrive over the long haul. Leaders use influence to shape the minds of followers; they elicit consent through persuasion, inspiration, and commitment. It is difficult for a single person to perform the roles of both management and leadership simultaneously because the two may have complementary strengths or require juggling conflicting agendas. Leadership and management function in dissimilar ways for the same goal of organizational success; however, both skill sets are needed for successful collaboration. Balanced leadership is essential, and earning the trust of internal and external stakeholders is important for implementing successful alignment strategies. This is one of the reasons that dyad leadership can be a practical solution to the challenges of the healthcare sector.

In their *Harvard Business Review* article "The Five Minds of a Manager," Jonathan Gosling and Henry Mintzberg (2003) suggest that employees no longer aspire to be a "good manager"—everybody wants to be a "great leader." To be effective, managers should focus not only on what they must accomplish, but also how they think.

Those two aspects establish the bounds of management: action and reflection. Action without reflection is thoughtless; reflection without action is passive. Every manager has to find a way to combine these two mind-sets—to function at the point where reflective thinking meets practical doing.

But action and reflection about what? One answer is collaboration—in negotiations, for example, where a manager cannot act alone. Action, reflection, and collaboration have to be rooted in a deep understanding of reality in all its facets. All three must be characterized by a certain analytical rationality or logic. Gosling and Mintzberg refer to this mind-set as *worldly*, which the Oxford English Dictionary defines as "experienced in life, sophisticated, practical."

FRAMEWORK AXES

Two interconnected axes form the framework used in this book: internal/external and flexibility/control. The first axis (internal/external) differentiates two important management considerations: centralized control (responsible for attaining high consistency and reliability of internal operations and organizational structures) and the development of strategies to adapt to rapid change in the business environment with flexibility. This dimension also relates to the strategy–structure congruence principle described in chapter 1. The pursuit of a sustained growth strategy (in exhibit 3.1, referred to as *scale*) depends on the ability of the organization to align its resources and capabilities (*build*) and even communication roles and skills (*develop*) with its larger community through engagement and innovative services (*innovate*).

As an example, most health systems strive to align clinical practices and services *internally* to ensure that the system operates reliably. The *external* goal of meeting community health needs is achieved by aligning organizational goals with the needs and interests of stakeholders (e.g., patient populations, health plans, employers, suppliers), complying effectively with laws and regulation, and maintaining robust financial performance. To fulfill its maximum potential, the organization must create sustainable linkages between clinical integration (which is internal) and community needs (which are external)—doing so facilitates patients' access to preventive and chronic care services and improves patient safety and quality (see also chapter 16).

The second axis of the framework (flexibility/control) reflects two important orientations of management philosophy: humanistic and rationalistic. The humanistic approach (represented by the upper half of exhibit 3.1) relies on interactive processes of communication, consultation, and involvement in decision-making and is typically associated with leadership. Leaders promote teamwork, self-direction, interfunctional collaboration, and joint accountability. They encourage teams to meet broad, emerging goals.

The rationalistic approach (represented by the lower half of exhibit 3.1) relies on centralized control and top-down communication, expecting employees and work groups to meet predetermined objectives. It is generally associated with the role of manager. Managers focus on fine-tuning structures and processes, achieving consistency and higher operating efficiency, applying proven solutions to problems, setting performance targets, monitoring implementation, and tracking results. While these two management philosophies, rationalistic and humanistic, seem mutually exclusive, when they converge, they create a balanced approach useful for dealing with the complexity inherent in the healthcare environment.

An organization's relative emphasis on the two philosophies reflects its own unique culture. In this chapter, and throughout the book, I will use the framework to demonstrate how dyads evolve with distinct configurations that incorporate overlapping management and leadership roles and responsibilities.

CONTEXT AND ROLES

When juxtaposed, the internal/external and flexibility/control axes create four target areas (population health, financial performance, clinical integration, patient engagement). Collectively, the dyad roles (health innovator, value strategist, clinical integration champion, patient advocate) and target areas cover many aspects of hospital performance management (see exhibit 3.2). The specific roles and responsibilities, however, vary based on the organizational size, complexity, department, service line, and hierarchical level in which the dyad operates.

The framework illustrates the dynamic tension between internal control and external flexibility and the advantages of having a broader, contextual view of the healthcare environment in responding to organizational challenges. An important condition for the

Exhibit 3.2: Dyads in Health Systems

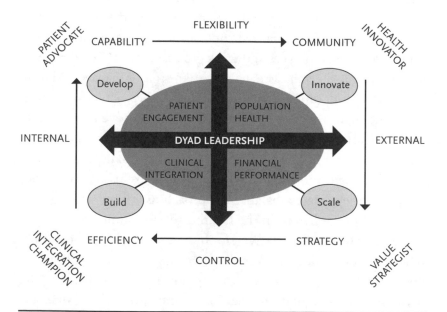

successful functioning of dyads involves the effective management of this tension.

ORGANIZING SCHEMA

Exhibit 3.3 describes the overlapping leadership roles for leading complex health systems: health innovator, value strategist, clinical integration champion, and patient advocate. Exhibit 3.4 reorganizes these same leadership roles and responsibilities, outlining which duties might be shared by a dyad of physician and administrator, as well as which duties might be exclusive to either role. As you examine exhibit 3.4, you can begin to imagine the relevance of the integrated approach and dyad leadership for responding effectively to the contradictory expectations and diverse stakeholders in the complex environment of healthcare systems.

Exhibit 3.3: Healthcare Leadership Target Areas and Responsibilities

Target Areas	Responsibilities
Population Health	Health Innovator
	• Redesigning health system services for population health
	• Improving care quality and patient safety
	• Reducing total cost of care for a population by fostering innovation
	• Catering to community needs
	• Promoting a culture of safety and reliability
	• Excelling in patient care with teamwork and innovative solutions
	• Improving care coordination and communication among clinicians, patients, and patients' families
	• Initiating referral relationships with hospitals in the accountable care organization (ACO)
	• Creating partnerships along the continuum of care to increase service lines
	• Developing formal partnerships and revamping or restructuring existing partnerships for an ACO contract

(continued)

Exhibit 3.3: Healthcare Leadership Target Areas and Responsibilities *(continued)*

Financial Performance	Value Strategist
	• Increasing scale by forming clinically integrated provider networks (formal, affiliated) and care systems • Expanding market share for ambulatory surgery centers and outpatient procedures • Reducing risk and promoting higher rates of utilization • Creating new service lines and revenue streams to increase profitability • Recruiting physicians to support growth and patient loyalty • Managing provider productivity • Strengthening finances to facilitate reinvestment and innovation implementation • Applying balanced scorecard • Conducting strategic analysis of competitors • Developing strategic planning and implementation • Monitoring internal supply chain performance • Managing human capital, staffing, and recruiting plans • Evaluating market share performance • Evaluating accounting and information systems and methods
Clinical Integration	**Clinical Integration Champion**
	• Integrating information technology (IT) systems • Implementing an electronic health record (EHR) • Optimizing clinical integration, aligned with a values-based culture • Improving interprofessional collaboration • Promoting teamwork among physicians and diverse care teams • Shaping the medical group practice culture • Improving cost containment and efficiency • Using analytics to improve coordination of care • Incorporating evidence-based information into patient diagnosis and treatment • Increasing the rate of interoperability of EHR systems to improve quality and reduce cost • Evaluating clinical outcomes • Supporting continuing education and skill development for clinical staff • Encouraging clinical care innovation

(continued)

Exhibit 3.3: Healthcare Leadership Target Areas and Responsibilities *(continued)*

Patient Engagement	Patient Advocate
	• Engaging physicians and patients in lowering clinical variation • Improving teamwork training and interpersonal skill building • Reducing readmissions • Tracking patient compliance with evidence-based practices • Increasing patient satisfaction and quality outcomes • Improving doctor–patient communication • Enhancing hospital credibility

Exhibit 3.4: Distributed and Shared Roles

Target: *Population Health* Role: *Health Innovator*		
Administrator	**Shared**	**Physician**
Reducing total cost of care for a population by fostering innovation	Redesigning health system services for population health	Improving care quality and patient safety
Creating partnerships along the continuum of care to increase service lines	Catering to community needs	Excelling in patient care with teamwork and innovative solutions
Developing formal partnerships (established to pursue an ACO contract), revamping or restructuring existing partnerships for an ACO contract	Promoting a culture of safety and reliability	Improving care coordination and communication among clinicians, patients, and patients' families

(continued)

Exhibit 3.4: Distributed and Shared Roles *(continued)*

	Creating partnerships along the continuum of care to increase variety and promote reliability
	Initiating referral relationships with hospitals in the ACO

**Target: *Financial Performance*
Role: *Value Strategist***

Administrator	Shared	Physician
Increasing scale by forming clinically integrated provider networks (formal, affiliated) and care systems	Expanding market share for ambulatory surgery centers (ASCs) and outpatient procedures	Reducing risk and promoting higher rates of utilization
Applying balanced scorecard	Managing provider productivity	Recruiting physicians to support growth and patient loyalty
Conducting competitor strategic analysis	Managing staffing and recruiting plans	
Monitoring internal supply chain performance	Developing strategic planning and implementation	
Evaluating market share performance	Managing human capital	
Evaluating accounting and information systems and methods	Creating new service lines and revenue streams to increase profitability	

(continued)

Exhibit 3.4: Distributed and Shared Roles *(continued)*

Strengthening finances to facilitate reinvestment and innovation implementation		

Target: *Clinical Integration* Role: *Clinical Integration Champion*		
Administrator	**Shared**	**Physician**
Integrating IT systems	Implementing EHRs	Optimizing clinical integration aligned with value-based culture
Improving cost containment and efficiency	Increasing the rate of interoperability to improve quality and reduce cost	Improving inter-professional collaboration
	Using analytics to improve coordination of care	Incorporating evidence-based information into patient diagnosis and treatment
	Complying with The Joint Commission's standards for clinical practice guidelines and quality control, and with Centers for Medicare & Medicaid Services regulation	Evaluating clinical outcomes
		Shaping the medical group practice culture

(continued)

Exhibit 3.4: Distributed and Shared Roles *(continued)*

		Promoting teamwork among physicians and diverse care teams
		Supporting physician continuing education and skill building
		Encouraging clinical care innovation

Target: *Patient Engagement*
Role: *Patient Advocate*

Administrator	Shared	Physician
Providing resources for training and development	Reducing readmissions	Engaging physicians and patients in lowering clinical variation
Enhancing hospital credibility	Improving teamwork training and interpersonal skill building	Tracking patient compliance with evidence-based practices
		Increasing patient satisfaction and quality outcomes
		Improving doctor–patient communication

Dyads use joint thinking, creative solutions to problems, and flexible behaviors to adapt to change. At the same time, they rely on more traditional, common methods of operations and practices to execute plans and enhance consistency.

KEY TAKEAWAYS

- The integrated approach to dyad leadership helps to link clinical integration and patient advocacy (internal concerns) with community needs and hospital performance (external concerns) and provides important insights about safety and quality.
- The humanistic and rationalistic approaches to leadership, when used together, create a synergistic, balanced approach useful for dealing with complexity.
- The dyad roles (health innovator, value strategist, clinical integration champion, patient advocate) and target areas (population health, financial performance, clinical integration, patient engagement) cover many aspects of hospital performance management.
- Dyad roles and target areas are interdependent, making the effects of shared leadership stronger.

REFERENCES

Belasen, A. T. 2008. *The Theory and Practice of Corporate Communication: A Competing Values Perspective*. Thousand Oaks, CA: SAGE Publications.

Belasen, A., B. Eisenberg, and J. Huppertz. 2015. *Mastering Leadership: A Vital Resource for Healthcare Organizations*. Burlington, MA: Jones & Bartlett Learning.

Cameron, K. S., and R. E. Quinn. 2006. *Diagnosing and Changing Organizational Culture: Based on the Competing Values Framework*. San Francisco: Jossey-Bass.

Gosling, J., and H. Mintzberg. 2003. "The Five Minds of a Manager." *Harvard Business Review*. Published November. https://hbr.org/2003/11/the-five-minds-of-a-manager.

CHAPTER 4

Dyad Roles: Self-Assessment

INTRODUCTION

This chapter introduces a self-administered questionnaire and a scoring method that will help you analyze the strengths and weaknesses of partners in a dyad. Self-assessments are essential for self-improvement. They are useful for ensuring that administrators and physicians achieve development and learning goals. When you and your coleader perform these assessments consecutively, they can provide a powerful image of how well you complement each other over time. You can also use your self-assessment to tailor training and improvement efforts to your needs, strengthening particular areas that are weak for you or your dyad.

Subsequent chapters will discuss specific examples and ways to strengthen the value proposition of the dyad. Future sections of the book also includes guidelines and examples of how to apply this assessment as a developmental tool for continuous improvement purposes.

GATHERING AND REPRESENTING INFORMATION

The first step in the objective analysis of your dyad is information gathering. Exhibit 4.1 shows a survey designed to gauge participants' primary responsibilities. These responsibilities are distributed across four sections, each reflecting the four dyad roles described in the previous chapter: health innovator (working in population health), value strategist (working in financial performance), CI champion (working in clinical integration, or CI), and patient advocate (working in patient engagement). Respondents consider each statement and use a seven-point scale to score how well it fits with their daily responsibilities and overall professional strengths.

Exhibit 4.1: Dyad Evaluation Survey

Frequency Level (Seven-Point Likert Scale)
Next to each statement indicate the response that best matches your situation. Make sure to mark your designated role: administrator (AD) or physician (MD).

1 — *Never*
2 — *Rarely (in fewer than 10 percent of my chances)*
3 — *Occasionally (in about 30 percent of my chances)*
4 — *Sometimes (in about 50 percent of my chances)*
5 — *Frequently (in about 70 percent of my chances)*
6 — *Usually (in about 90 percent of my chances)*
7 — *Every time*

Population Health (Health Innovator)

	AD	MD
1. I pursue an ACO contract or revamp existing partnerships for an ACO contract.		
2. I consider an investment in population health analytics to be a high priority.		
3. I use analytics to help measure performance across cost and quality measures.		
4. I promote the use of electronic health records (EHRs) and health information technology to improve safety across the continuum of care.		
5. I initiate data sharing with ancillary providers.		

(continued)

Exhibit 4.1: Dyad Evaluation Survey *(continued)*

6. I initiate improvement in safety and best practice–sharing among ACOs.

7. I track the attainment of the Triple Aim.

8. I view a problem through the patient's perspective rather than that of the provider or the institution.

9. I initiate collaboration among sector partners, technology developers, healthcare leaders, clinicians, and patients to increase safety and reliability.

10. I use needs assessment to identify potential innovations.

11. I secure sustainable funding to implement innovations.

12. I find ways to reduce total cost of care for a population by fostering innovation.

13. I work with hospital partners to leverage resources to improve community health.

14. I spur collaboration between providers and patients across the entire continuum of care to reduce cost.

15. I promote a culture of safety and reliability in my health system.

Financial Performance (Value Strategist)

	AD	MD
16. I focus on balancing my healthcare system's revenues and expenses.		
17. I monitor excess margins, operating margins, and patient care margins.		
18. I ensure that adequate capital is available to deliver services.		

(continued)

Exhibit 4.1: Dyad Evaluation Survey *(continued)*

19. I secure sufficient capital capacity and access for short and long-term operations.

20. I make sure that my healthcare system has the resources to renew itself.

21. I maintain higher margins and cash flow to help finance expansion plans.

22. I work to expand market share for ambulatory surgery centers in areas where my health system does not own or operate acute care hospitals.

23. I create opportunities for new service lines and revenue streams to increase profitability.

24. I use the balanced scorecard (BSC) to monitor the attainment of strategic goals.

25. I use the BSC to review how we look to our stakeholders.

26. I conduct competitor strategic analysis using benchmarking methods.

27. I engage in strategic planning and implementation.

28. I monitor internal supply chain performance.

29. I evaluate market share performance.

30. I initiate a turnaround strategy in recruiting and retention of physicians to increase my hospital's referral base.

Clinical Integration (CI Champion)

	AD	MD
31. I strengthen the strategic alignment between the CI network and other partners within the health system.		
32. I monitor the implementation of EHRs.		
33. I ensure that clinical integration aligns with the hospital's value-based culture.		

(continued)

Exhibit 4.1: Dyad Evaluation Survey *(continued)*

34. I develop plans for improving interprofessional collaboration.

35. I initiate an increase in the rate of interoperability to improve quality and reduce cost.

36. I help shape the medical group practice culture.

37. I devise plans for improving cost containment and efficiency.

38. I facilitate the coordination of patient care across providers.

39. I use analytics to improve coordination of care.

40. I encourage clinical care innovation across my provider networks and care systems.

41. I support continuing education and skill development for clinicians.

42. I develop opportunities for physician groups, healthcare systems, and other entities to work together to provide comprehensive coverage for an entire market.

43. I focus on care improvement for all patients who access the network.

44. I develop financial incentives to support the goals of clinical integration.

45. I look for opportunities to work together with other providers to maximize efficiencies and provide a better overall experience to the patient.

Patient Engagement (Patient Advocate)

	AD	MD
46. I treat patients with courtesy and respect.		
47. I listen carefully to patients.		
48. I keep eye contact with my patients.		

(continued)

49. I focus on the patient to help reduce hospital readmission.

50. I encourage assessment and development of emotional intelligence and interpersonal skills of care team members.

51. I monitor patient wait time.

52. I promote patient safety through teamwork.

53. I do everything to help patients with pain management treatment.

54. I find out new ways of documenting clinical encounters and using data.

55. I explain possible side effects in a way that patients understand.

56. I include the patient's family members in consultations.

57. I encourage professional communication and spur collaborative team efforts.

58. I follow up with patients upon discharge to improve medication adherence.

59. I place great emphasis on the cleanliness and tidiness of hospital rooms.

60. I use various media to increase patients' meaningful participation.

We can see the value of the assessment instrument through the example of a senior-level dyad at a hospital located in New England. The coleaders are an executive vice president/chief operating officer (AD) and an executive vice president/system chief medical officer (MD). The histogram in exhibit 4.2 shows the dyad's survey results. While the physician's strengths lie in the roles of patient advocate

Exhibit 4.2: Relative Strengths of Administrator–Physician Dyad

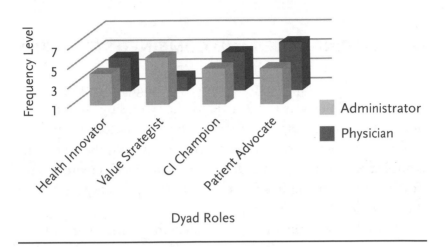

and CI champion, the administrator's strengths are associated with the value strategist and health innovator roles.

DYAD ASSESSMENT: OVERCOMING BLIND SPOTS

More sophisticated assessments of the dyad's survey results can be generated using a simple Excel spreadsheet, converted into a more digestible visual format. This chapter uses an image called a radar chart (also sometimes called a spider chart), which makes patterns instantly visible. Radar charts (or spidergrams) are helpful for comparing multiple quantitative variables on axes that have the same starting point. Axes are arranged outwardly, with equal distances and the same scale between all axes. Each variable value is plotted along its individual axis and connected together to form a polygon. They are useful for seeing which variables are scoring relatively high or low in a data set, making them ideal for visualizing leadership roles and competencies or conducting gap analysis.

OVERLAPPING ROLES AND COMBINED STRENGTHS

Exhibit 4.3 is a radar chart of the New England dyad's survey responses. It illustrates the fact that although a single leader does not possess the full capacity to meet the expectations in the four key areas, if they work as a pair (see exhibit 4.4), the coleaders' complementary strengths cover most of their task environment. This combined strength is what makes the dyad indispensable for the success of the organization.

When the role strengths are combined, the partners respond well to the requirements in their task environment (exhibit 4.4). The values

---

Exhibit 4.3: Dyad Leadership at Senior-Level Management

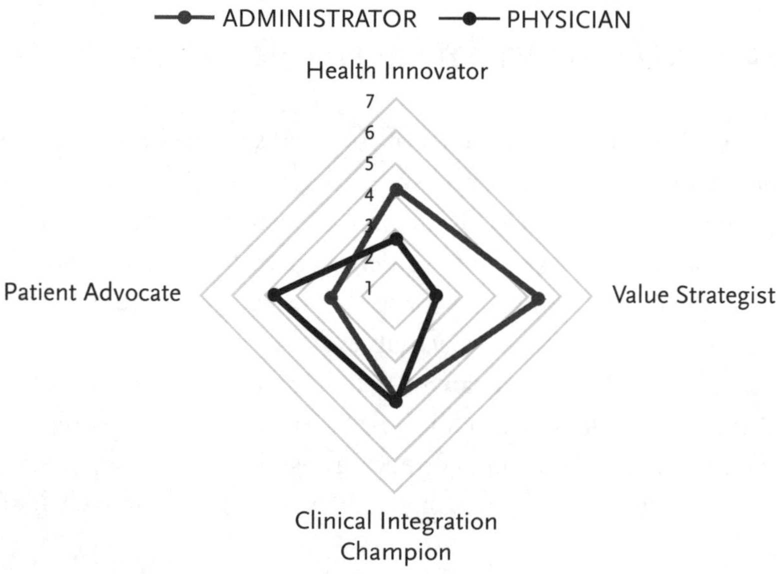

ADMINISTRATOR   PHYSICIAN

Health Innovator

7
6
5
4
3
2
1

Patient Advocate

Value Strategist

Clinical Integration
Champion

Exhibit 4.4: Combined Strengths of the Dyad Across the Roles

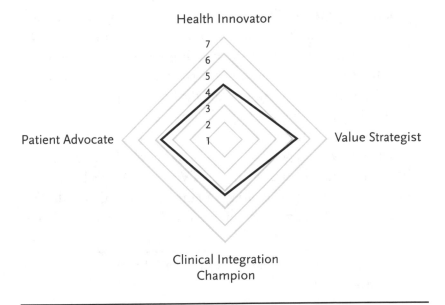

in exhibit 4.4 represent the average ratings for each role played by the dyad. Their complementary roles and skills create a synergistic effect that helps mitigate their relative weaknesses or blind spots in the low-scoring areas of the dyad. Through learning and further education and development, the combined profile of the dyad can be expanded for optimal performance. To determine the most important areas for improvement, the partners can review, discuss, and compare their scores for each role. They can identify weak spots and sweet spots for further development and mutually agree on improvement efforts that can further optimize their collaborative efforts.

The dyad's development plans, skill building, and improvement efforts should preferably match the health system's strategic goals and future directions. Thus, the assessment serves as a powerful way to link leadership roles and competencies with present and future organizational goals and strategies.

COMPARING RELATIVE STRENGTHS

By comparing the dyad's responses to survey questions intended to measure their abilities as health innovators, exhibit 4.5 visually represents their responses to the health population section of the survey. In health systems, health innovators focus on enhancing the patient experience of care, improving the health of populations, and reducing the per capita cost of healthcare.

Increasing patient safety is a good example of the duties of a health innovator, and both ADs and MDs have much to contribute to improvement. Creating a culture of safety requires a leader with the mind-set of a high-reliability organization—a figure who can transcend specialized areas and empower staff members to collaborate

Exhibit 4.5: Population Health and Health Innovator Complementary Roles

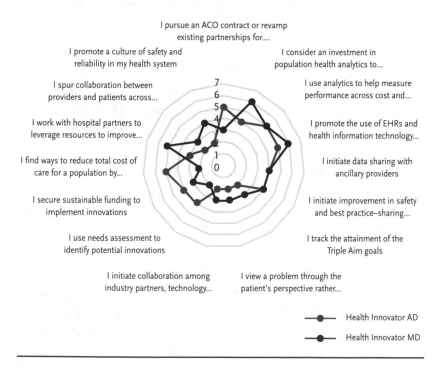

in identifying possible failures and tackling them innovatively and responsibly. Good leaders model the way to safety by walking the talk and by giving employees the right tools and resources to be successful. Promoting a culture of safety is reinforced through a commitment to transparent communications in response to adverse events, near misses, and unsafe conditions.

Exhibit 4.6 maps out the New England hospital dyad's capacity in the field of financial management, as the two partners to the dyad try to fulfill the role of value strategist. For example, the recruitment of new physicians and support staff, while important for physicians, is initiated primarily by administrators. Strategic planning and attempts to expand market share, while not a traditional area of focus for physicians (see exhibit 4.6), requires their support and consultation.

Exhibit 4.7 illustrates that while clinical decisions are the purview of physicians, and while administrators influence planning and coordination, the partners in our hospital dyad seem to complement

---

Exhibit 4.6: Financial Management and Value Strategist Complementary Roles

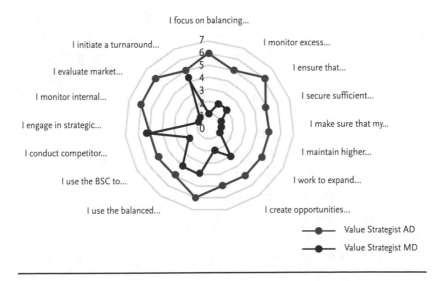

Exhibit 4.7: Clinical Integration and CI Champion Complementary Roles

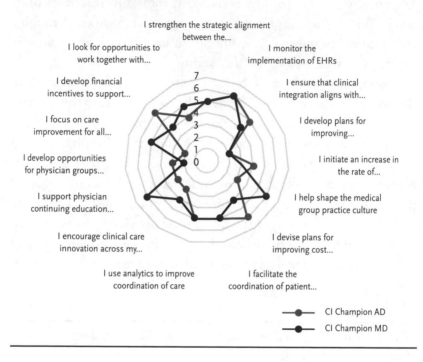

each other relatively well in the role of CI champion. In general, physicians display strengths in the east-and-west side of the framework and administrators in the north-and-south. Together, the coleaders work to reduce variation and the propensity for failure by promoting clinical integration and by cherishing mutual respect, trust, and teamwork.

Exhibit 4.8 analyzes the abilities of our doctor and administrator as they perform the role of health advocate. While the patient engagement inherent in health advocacy would seem to be the province of the doctor–patient relationship, in reality, its foundation is built by administrators (see exhibit 4.8). For example, it is imperative that hospital administrators stress open and clear communication between doctors and patients to avoid a range of problems that

Exhibit 4.8: Patient Engagement and Health Advocacy Complementary Roles

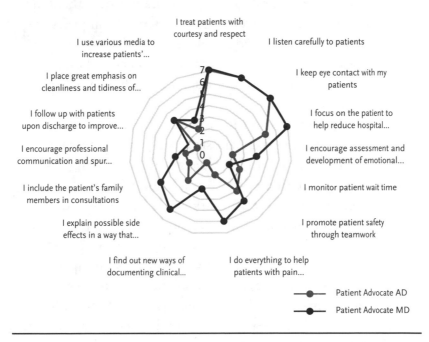

I treat patients with courtesy and respect
I use various media to increase patients'...
I listen carefully to patients
I place great emphasis on cleanliness and tidiness of...
I keep eye contact with my patients
I follow up with patients upon discharge to improve...
I focus on the patient to help reduce hospital...
I encourage professional communication and spur...
I encourage assessment and development of emotional...
I include the patient's family members in consultations
I monitor patient wait time
I explain possible side effects in a way that...
I promote patient safety through teamwork
I find out new ways of documenting clinical...
I do everything to help patients with pain...

Patient Advocate AD
Patient Advocate MD

affect the organization as a whole. Patients who report positive communication with their doctors are likely to communicate pertinent information about their ailments more quickly and will be more likely to adhere to treatment regimens, improving outcomes and satisfaction scores—all matters of concern to administrators. While doctors may need training to supplement or alter their standard "script" when communicating with patients, this investment of time and funds will inevitably be worth the cost.

Sometimes, however, the perceptual gaps between how healthcare leaders view the effectiveness of their organizations versus how physicians believe they perform their communicative duties versus how patients feel are too wide to overcome. Mismatches such as these will be discussed in subsequent chapters.

KEY TAKEAWAYS

- The charts in exhibits 4.2, 4.3, and 4.4 illustrate that, on balance, the administrator–physician dyad comprises the synergistic abilities and strengths demanded by the four key areas of hospital management: population health, financial performance, clinical integration, and patient engagement.
- You can use similar charts to demonstrate the efficacy of your dyad management structure by assessing your personal strengths and weaknesses and identifying potential gaps or areas for further improvement.
- Others at the same organization may also complete the assessment, including any combination of team members, peers, and supervisors. The objective is to provide a more accurate measure of gaps between what healthcare leaders say about themselves and how others evaluate them.
- If the ratings from the self-assessment match the ratings from others, they serve to confirm that the partners in the dyad perform their roles well within expectations.
- If the differences are significant, they provide important insights about key areas that require fine-tuning. The partners in the dyad can focus on the areas with the greatest gaps and prioritize their training and development efforts.
- Over time, the assessment can serve as a powerful tool for self-development and continuous improvement.

PART II

Role: Health Innovator

Exhibit 2: Health Innovator

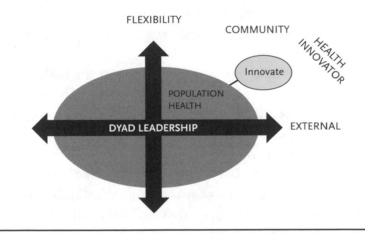

In 2007, the Institute for Healthcare Improvement (IHI) articulated three overarching goals, called the *Triple Aim*, for quality improvement. Hospitals that want to provide quality care should consider all three goals simultaneously (IHI 2019):

1. Improving the patient experience of care (including quality and satisfaction)
2. Improving the health of populations
3. Reducing the per capita cost of healthcare

The central focus of the Triple Aim is on improving the delivery of care to individuals and families, transforming the role of primary care, maintaining the health of populations, reducing cost, and harnessing the power and possibility of information technology. These goals are essential components of the continuum of care, which integrates medicine, public health, and social services.

The new approach is introspective in a sense that upstream problems and solutions are identified proactively to reduce the potential for medical errors, miscommunications, and hospital readmissions. Among leaders, successful outcomes require a willingness to take on new roles and commit to honest self-appraisal. In turn, the per capita cost of care is expected to stabilize and even be reduced. Meeting the Triple Aim will help to ensure downstream caregiving, providing equitable access to services and wellness and sustaining the overall goals of increased value.

Achieving the Triple Aim is the basic goal for the health innovator role of the dyad as leaders address population health costs and quality care issues. To more fully explore that role, chapter 5 covers its context, with a primary focus on enhancing the patient experience—the first part of the Triple Aim—by reducing medical errors, monitoring unnecessary readmissions, and increasing safety through innovation. Chapter 6 centers on improving health populations, the second of the IHI's goals, through a wide variety of means, including stakeholder inclusion, effective use of evidence-based practices, and technological innovation. Chapter 7 examines issues relating to risk management and cost control, in concert with the third prong of the Triple Aim. Chapter 8 extends the discussion to types of accountable care organizations, bundled payments, and risk stratification, as well as developing meaningful collaborative efforts with community agencies and the public health system. Chapter 9 concludes part II with a discussion of innovation and cultural transformation.

REFERENCE

Institute for Healthcare Improvement. 2019. "IHI Triple Aim Initiative." Accessed January 16. www.ihi.org/engage/initiatives/TripleAim/Pages/default.aspx.

CHAPTER 5

The Context for the Dyad Health Innovator

INTRODUCTION

Achieving the goals of the Triple Aim—improving the patient experience of care, improving the health of populations, and reducing per capita healthcare costs—requires a commitment to interprofessional collaboration, a culture of safety and innovation, and teamwork. In addition to aligning quality goals and incentives, harnessing innovation technology, and embracing evidence-based medicine, dyad leaders in the capacity of health innovator can initiate partnerships and model the way forward to members of their organization. Health innovators use fresh thinking on innovation and quality, and they seek to transform the culture of the organization.

IMPROVING THE PATIENT EXPERIENCE

According to the Agency for Healthcare Research and Quality (AHRQ 2018), health systems have significantly reduced the rate of hospital-acquired conditions (HAC)—problems a patient develops while being treated in the hospital for a different clinical issue. In part as a result of the Affordable Care Act (ACA), an estimated 125,000 fewer patients died as a result of HACs in 2010–2015, and more than $28 billion in savings was accrued during that period. Exhibit 5.1 shows that, cumulatively, approximately 3.1 million fewer incidents of harm occurred between 2011 and 2015 (compared with 2010) (AHRQ 2016). In total, hospital patients experienced a decline of 21 percent in the rate of adverse effects (exhibit 5.2). Health innovators working at organizations across the country have contributed to these major improvements. Dyad leaders everywhere can learn from similarly groundbreaking measures taken in many sectors of the field, not just hospitals, to bring about improvements in areas of need.

The decline results in part from the ACA's push to improve the quality of healthcare by aligning Centers for Medicare & Medicaid

Exhibit 5.1: Total Annual and Cumulative Cost Savings (Compared With 2010 Baseline)

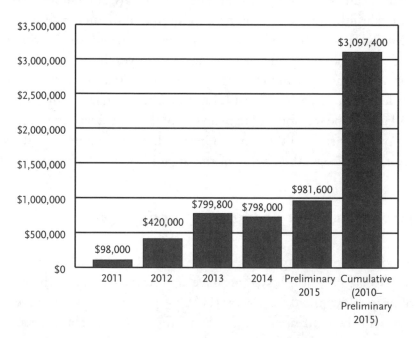

Source: AHRQ (2016).

Exhibit 5.2: Annual and Cumulative Changes in HACs, 2010–2015

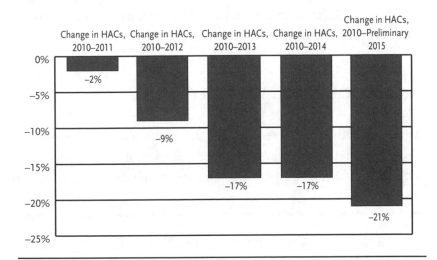

Source: AHRQ (2016).

Services (CMS) financial incentives with a focus on patient safety. However, other contributing factors, include the following:

- Public reporting of hospital-level results
- Technical assistance offered to hospitals by the Quality Improvement Organization (QIO)
- Technical assistance and increased efforts by the Department of Health and Human Services' Partnership for Patients initiative, led by CMS.

In addition to these efforts, AHRQ (2017) has developed a variety of methods, tools, and resources to help hospitals and other providers prevent HACs such as adverse drug events, catheter-associated urinary tract infections, pressure ulcers, surgical site infections, injuries, and falls.

The Mayo Center for Innovation, with its focus on transforming the patient experience and delivery of healthcare, relies on multidisciplinary teams to implement patient-centered innovation. Dyad leaders in the role of health innovator can benefit from learning about Mayo's innovation programs (see Mayo Clinic Center for Innovation).

CROWDSOURCING IN HEALTHCARE

With rapid advances in technology, improvements in telecommunication systems, and the expanded use of mobile devices, open innovation (OI), and crowdsourcing are taking on an increasingly

Mayo Clinic Center for Innovation: 58 Hospitals and Health Systems with Innovation Programs, 2017

Designers and administrators at the Mayo Clinic Center for Innovation aim to change healthcare delivery by focusing on the human experience to identify design needs. The center has collaborated with several Mayo departments on multiple innovation initiatives, including efforts to transform room design and a telemedicine program dubbed eConsults, which uses audiovisual technology for real-time patient–provider interactions and eliminates the need for in-person follow-up visits. Additionally, the center hosts an annual two-day healthcare innovation conference called Transform, which brings together providers, designers, entrepreneurs, and more to collaborate and share information that can help spur change in the healthcare delivery experience.

—*Becker's Hospital Review* (2017)

important role across many sectors—including healthcare. Getting input from people who use the healthcare system helps dyad leaders in the role of health innovators ensure effectiveness of outcomes.

Open Innovation

In OI, organizations solicit the help, input, and information of a variety of potential partners—including community groups and market share rivals. OI helps companies reduce the cost of product development and process improvement, minimize time to market for new products, improve product quality, and access customer and supplier expertise outside the organization. For OI to be successful, ideas must be shared both internally and externally through collaborative networks or partnerships.

AstraZeneca, an internationally known pharmaceutical company, embraces OI. Astra has spent the past few years forging partnerships with groups including health charities, academic researchers, and even competitor GlaxoSmithKline. The organizations share early-stage research, using the knowledge to solve particular disease problems. Often the process involves sharing labs with researchers from other organizations. According to Mene Pangalos, Astra's head of innovative medicines, "It enables us to get more out of our research dollars than by just doing things on our own. You're creating an ecosystem where you can collaborate and get more out of it than if you were just doing something on your own" (Roland 2014).

Another example is Cisco's Entrepreneurs in Residence, an incubation program that supports early-stage entrepreneurs who are working on projects that may benefit the organization (Anand 2014). Those selected receive financial support, industry expertise, and access to business groups. Program events include opportunities to present the ideas to investors and to work side by side with the experts at Cisco. This is advantageous for both parties—the entrepreneurs receive opportunity and support, and Cisco is able to bring in fresh minds and revolutionary ideas from outside of the company.

Crowdsourcing

Crowdsourced innovation happens when the expertise of a broad variety of volunteers is solicited online. Organizations may request help with developing insight or proposals, setting priorities, or even prototyping and evaluating new ideas. For example, Siemens Automation's user forum focuses on quality management. Contributors are encouraged to provide information; users rate the validity and usefulness of the information, then contributions are categorized.

Crowdsourcing is helping scientists collaborate on large-scale health projects, such as pandemics. One example of this is a Crowd-Med's online platform to which physicians post difficult cases to seek help from a secure, intimate group of colleagues. The platform can help doctors and health systems save time and money by directing doctors to appropriate solutions, reducing the number of unnecessary tests, ineffective treatments, and consultations.

CrowdMed charges patients a fee to list their case and receive input about a possible diagnosis. Patients fill out a patient questionnaire that details their symptoms, case history, and personal information. Once a case is posted, the crowd ("MDs" or "medical detectives") can review the patient's information and offer up what they believe is a likely diagnosis. Nearly 3,000 people have signed up as medical detectives, including doctors and residents (Strohmeyer 2013).

Webicina is a site where medicine combines with social media to allow physicians across the world to communicate their answers to health questions quickly and effectively. PatientsLikeMe allows individuals with certain health conditions to share and compare their symptoms and responses to different treatments. The site offers an Open Research Exchange platform that allows researchers to develop, test, and conduct surveys in the site's community of more than 200,000 members (Strohmeyer 2013).

PARTNERSHIP FOR PATIENTS

The Partnership for Patients (PfP) is a public–private partnership. Its participating groups of physicians, nurses, hospitals, employers, patients and their advocates, and the federal and state governments form networks that focus on making hospital care safer, more reliable, and less costly. They pursue two goals:

1. *Delivering safer care.* Keep patients from getting injured or sicker. Decrease all-cause patient harm by 20 percent compared to the 2014 interim baseline (121 HACs per 1,000 patient discharges).
2. *Improving care transitions.* Help patients heal without complications. Decrease preventable complications during a transition from one care setting to another. Reduce all 30-day hospital readmissions by 12 percent as a population-based measure (readmissions per 1,000 people) (CMS 2019).

Hospital Improvement Innovation Networks

On September 28, 2016, CMS awarded contracts to 16 Hospital Improvement Innovation Networks (HIINs) as a part of the integration of the PfP Hospital Engagement Networks (HEN) into the Quality Improvement Network–Quality Improvement Organization (QIN–QIO) program. Through the PfP, the 16 national, regional, or state hospital associations, quality improvement organizations, and health system organizations serve as HIINs. The HIINs also represent the integration of the work previously done by the HENs in support of the QIN–QIO and quality improvement efforts for the Medicare population.

Another major PfP network includes the 46 sites selected to participate in the Community-Based Care Transitions program. Each brings together community-based organizations such as social service providers, agencies on aging, multiple hospital partners, nursing homes, home health agencies, pharmacies, primary care practices, and other types of health and social service providers serving patients in that community. Through the program, these sites are testing models for improving care transitions from the hospital to other settings and for reducing readmissions for high-risk Medicare beneficiaries.

Communication among healthcare professionals, clinicians, and patients and their families is critical for the successful outcomes that health innovators pursue. It is a key part of keeping patients from getting injured or sicker in the hospital, helping patients heal without complication through improved transitions, and reducing readmissions.

KEY TAKEAWAYS

- The decline in the rate of harmful healthcare incidents in the United States aligns with a major goal of the ACA, defined previously to improve the quality of healthcare by aligning CMS financial incentives with a shared and sustained focus on patient safety.
- The PfP involves physicians, nurses, hospitals, employers, patients, and patient advocates, as well as federal and state governments.
- The cornerstone of reducing costs and improving the quality of care is making hospitals safer and more reliable.
- Open innovation and crowdsourcing provide access to the collective intelligence of a pool of experts to optimize treatment plans for patients.

REFERENCES

Agency for Healthcare Research and Quality (AHRQ). 2018. "AHRQ Scorecard on Hospital-Acquired Conditions." Reviewed

June. www.ahrq.gov/professionals/quality-patient-safety/pfp/index.html.

———.2017. "AHRQ Tools to Reduce Hospital-Acquired Conditions." Reviewed December. www.ahrq.gov/professionals/quality-patient-safety/hac/tools.html.

———. 2016. "National Scorecard on Rates of Hospital-Acquired Conditions 2010 to 2015: Interim Data from National Efforts to Make Health Care Safer." Reviewed December. www.ahrq.gov/professionals/quality-patient-safety/pfp/2015-interim.html.

Anand, M. 2014. "Launching Cisco Entrepreneurs in Residence in Europe." Cisco. Published July 22. https://blogs.cisco.com/news/launching-cisco-entrepreneurs-in-residence-in-europe.

Becker's Hospital Review. 2017. "Mayo Clinic Center for Innovation: 58 Hospitals and Health Systems with Innovation Programs 2017." Published September 28. www.beckershospitalreview.com/58-hospitals-and-health-systems-with-innovation-programs-2017/mayo-clinic-center-for-innovation-17.

Centers for Medicare & Medicaid Services (CMS). 2019. "About the Partnership for Patients." Accessed January 16. https://partnershipforpatients.cms.gov/about-the-partnership/aboutthepartnershipforpatients.html.

Roland, D. 2014. "AstraZeneca Reinforces Pipeline with 'Open Innovation.'" *Telegraph* (UK). Published April 28. www.telegraph.co.uk/finance/newsbysector/pharmaceuticalsandchemicals/10775160/AstraZeneca-reinforces-pipeline-with-open-innovation.html.

Strohmeyer, K. 2013. "Not Alone in a Crowd: Crowdsourcing for Healthcare." *Healthcare IT News.* Published July 9. www.healthcareitnews.com/blog/not-alone-crowd-crowdsourcing-healthcare.

CHAPTER 6

Improving the Health of Populations

INTRODUCTION

Population health integrates medicine, which focuses on treating individuals through the healthcare system, with public health services and interventions, which protect broader populations from illnesses and injury through the policies and programs. Although the benefits of population health strategies may be most visible in underserved communities or at safety net hospitals, health systems serving all types of communities should integrate this approach to achieve higher rates of effectiveness and efficiency.

Though population health is a desirable goal, its challenges are many. A single patient likely logs multiple episodes of care with various providers throughout a health system; therefore, attempts to improve the patient experience require extensive coordination across the continuum of care. Such coordination helps facilitate the best outcomes for patients—and the health of the population—and improves the quality of patient care.

Achieving population health does not stop at care coordination, however. Healthcare organizations should work to improve the ways in which they manage staff (e.g., engage leaders, inspire staff), develop strategy (e.g., risk stratify populations, measure variation in care), and empower patients. Chapter 6 discusses these efforts in depth.

TYPES OF POPULATION HEALTH

In healthcare, there are two common approaches to envisioning populations: discrete populations (also called *defined populations*) and regional populations (also called *community-based populations*) (Lewis 2014). Discrete populations are groups of individuals receiving care within a health system, or whose care is covered through a specific health plan or entity. Examples of a discrete population include employees of an organization, members of a health plan, the people included in a practice's patient panel, or all those enrolled in a particular accountable care organization (ACO).

Regional populations, on the other hand, are inclusive population segments, defined geographically. People in a segment of community population are identified by a common set of needs or issues, such as babies with low birth weight or older adults with complex needs. Unlike defined populations, however, these individuals may receive care from a variety of health systems or may be unconnected to care. They may or may not be insured. Individuals within a regional population are often difficult to count with a high level of certainty.

When they are acting as population health innovators, dyad leaders—working with other ACO partners—review their patient population and areas in which they will likely be able to make a measurable, meaningful impact on quality. The ACO must be willing to engage mission-driven clinics, practices, and partners who are committed to a culture of care and focused on achieving the Triple Aim. The ACO partners often initiate improvement in current capabilities of the health network, community-based partnerships, and methods of delivery. These may include the initiatives described in the following sections (Penso 2017).

MANAGING STAFF FOR POPULATION HEALTH

Engaging Leaders in Evidence-Based Practices

Health system leaders have a critical role in championing the quality improvements necessary to population health. To do so, effective leaders engage in evidence-based practices and conflict resolution, and they have negotiation skills that win stakeholder buy-in. Leaders must have patience, recognizing that capital investments in health information technology (IT), hiring, training and development, and cultural transformation may not have immediate payoffs. Investing time and energy in developing and engaging administrative and clinical leaders helps to sustain their learning curve.

Motivating Employees

Generating short-term wins as part of a process for linking positive outcomes with change helps dyad leaders facilitate strategy implementation. Winning is contagious. Everyone wants to associate themselves with successful outcomes. The foundation of high-level wins, however, is wise organizational goals that inspire staff. SMART goals are one useful technique, as they direct attention and energy to clear and reachable aims. For optimal employee engagement, make sure that the goals you set before your staff meet the following criteria:

- Specific
- Measurable
- Achievable
- Realistic
- Timely

By making the goals Specific, they can be Measurable. For example, instead of stating a goal like "improve quality of patient care," a more effective goal would be "reduce the 30-day readmissions rate by 75 percent," which is a very clear aim that all would agree is critical for the organization. The goal also has to be Achievable, and in this example, dyad leaders recognize that reducing 30-day readmissions by 75 percent might not be practical, since a great many factors lie outside the providers' control. Dyad leaders may *want* to reduce readmissions by 75 percent, but the goal must also be Realistic. Finally, goals must be Timely, a parameter that sets a relevant time frame for attaining the goal. A restated goal might be "within the next 12 months, reduce the 30-day readmissions rate by 25 percent."

Communicating Through Stories

Harnessing the power of imagination through stories, ceremonies, and symbols helps to engage team members and inspires commitment and collaboration. Leaders may initiate important events and ceremonies to celebrate team accomplishments and use storytelling and symbols, which are powerful media, to present ideas in a rich, colorful way that connects with members on impact. Dyad leaders communicate through success stories and encourage members to embrace the new discourse about value-based care and population health. Identifying positive role models and champions of change to inspire others helps lower resistance and increase cooperation.

STRATEGIZING FOR POPULATION HEALTH

Improving Analytics

Health systems have spent many years and a considerable amount of money on implementing electronic health records, but we haven't really reaped the benefits of data analytics or increased productivity.

Dyad health innovators collaborate with IT experts and clinicians to design and implement analytics with the goal of reducing unnecessary inefficiencies and administrative costs, upgrading care coordination, and improving patient wellness. These innovations are within reach, and they are a necessary component of population health.

Creating Effective Care Teams

A team approach among clinicians is critical to achieving the high-quality healthcare from which population health arises. Strong evidence indicates that primary care practices benefit from employing a team-based model of collaboration, wherein care teams explicitly share responsibility for a defined group of patients and have resources to support team-based care. Team-based care coordination also lowers hospital and emergency room (ER) admissions and reduces operating costs for health systems. It boosts nurse retention, increases patient satisfaction, and improves the overall patient experience (*Becker's Hospital Review* 2013a).

Risk Stratification

A vital part of improving the overall health of a population, and of bringing down costs while improving quality, is targeting the sickest patients for intensive support. Proactively identifying your high-cost subpopulation by targeting the drivers of excess utilization is crucial for maintaining financial success. In general, a small percentage of patients (usually those with complex or multiple medical conditions who are likely to incur high costs and experience poor outcomes) account for the majority of healthcare spending. One effective way of dealing with the challenges such patients pose is to structure population health programs through the management of high-risk care. A patient-centric approach, which directs additional resources and services toward the chronically ill, could substantially reduce costs and improve quality.

Involving Stakeholders from the Start

Effective population health strategies extend beyond the current episode-based framework of patient care to involve a variety of stakeholders. Considerable engagement among the ACO partners, affiliated doctors, hospitals, and other healthcare providers as they review and agree on expectations is vital for building a successful population health program.

Communication from the start is key—health systems must involve the right personnel at the right clinic sites at the right times. To ensure seamless transition of patients from one clinic site to another, the planning process must include a clear delineation of the roles and responsibilities of all care team members. These include clinical staff, behavioral health providers, pharmacists, nurses, call center staff, laboratory department personnel, nursing home administrators, and frontline office staff.

Assigning Patients to Primary Care

Primary care shifts the focus from physician-centered care to patient-centered care and is the backbone of population health. Assigning each patient to a primary care physician or care team is essential for achieving successful outcomes, including high-quality care, patient satisfaction, and efficient use of resources. An increase of one primary care doctor per 10,000 people has been shown to result in the following:

- 5 percent decrease in outpatient visits
- 5.5 percent decrease in inpatient admissions
- 10.9 percent decrease in ER visits
- 7.2 percent decrease in surgeries (American Academy of Family Physicians 2019)

Measuring Variation in Care

Understanding and managing clinical variation is essential for measuring efficiency and effectiveness within a population. It also helps drive quality and reduce cost. While some variation in care is normal, measuring how differences in clinical processes result in differences in quality and costs is important—only then can healthcare organizations address their opportunities for improvement.

POPULATION HEALTH THROUGH EMPOWERING PATIENTS

At the heart of population health is the patient. Empowering patients, and actively engaging them in the decision-making process, establishes an environment of trust, promotes patient centeredness, and ultimately increases patient satisfaction. Healthcare organizations must enable patients to become partners in their care; doing so allows the organization to identify the solutions that are working from the patient's perspective. When patient empowerment is carried out well, patients participate more fully and actively and leave the hospital with an enhanced motivation to adhere to care management requirements.

Disruptive Innovation in Healthcare: Examples from 3 Top Health Systems

[Colorado-based health system Catholic Health Initiatives (CHI)] has created a new infrastructure for the delivery of healthcare that shifts the central focus from the acute-care hospital to outpatient facilities and the home. . . . Focusing on outpatient care and care closer to home signals a shift from only treating sick patients to preventing sickness and maintaining people's health in addition to treating sick patients.

We're organizing our physicians, hospitals, and ambulatory healthcare delivery network providers into a more rational system. We're not waiting for people to become patients to serve them; we're establishing more robust relationships in our communities to help people achieve and maintain their care while ensuring that essential medical care is delivered in the most appropriate settings—even when that means arranging for care outside our hospitals and specialist services.

One of the keys to this new infrastructure is access to more data on patients, allowing providers to manage population health. CHI can monitor care ranging from primary settings to ERs to specific service lines.

Another disruptive innovation at CHI is an orientation toward patients as consumers and a greater connection between the system and community. "We are moving into a customer relationship management phase, investing time and energy resources in connecting with our patients and with consumers who are part of either employer groups or other defined populations that subscribe to our health system."

—*Becker's Hospital Review* (2013b)

KEY TAKEAWAYS

- As they work toward population health, health system leaders have a critical role in championing quality improvements and investing in long-term goals.
- SMART goals provide greater focus and direct attention and energy to clear and reachable goals.
- Dyad health innovators, IT experts, and clinicians collaborate in the design and implementation of data analytics innovations to improve process outcomes.
- Team-based care coordination lowers hospital and emergency room admissions and reduces operating costs.
- Primary care shifts the focus from physician-centered care to patient-centered care and is the backbone of population health.
- Healthcare leaders should enable patients to become partners in their care and learn from them what is working.

REFERENCES

American Academy of Family Physicians. 2019. "Why Primary Care Matters." Accessed February 6. www.aafp.org/medical-school -residency/choosing-fm/value-scope.html.

Becker's Hospital Review. 2013a. "Advanced Medical Teams: Improving Patient Health, Care Coordination at Iowa Health." Published February 8. www.beckershospitalreview.com/hospital -physician-relationships/advanced-medical-teams-improving -patient-health-care-coordination-at-iowa-health.html.

―――. 2013b. "Disruptive Innovation in Healthcare: Examples from 3 Top Health Systems." Published January 11. www. beckershospitalreview.com/strategic-planning/disruptive- innovation-in-healthcare-examples-from-3-top-health-systems. html.

Lewis, N. 2014. "Populations, Population Health, and the Evolution of Population Management: Making Sense of the Terminology in US Health Care Today." Institute for Healthcare Improvement. Published March 19. www.ihi.org/communities/blogs/population-health-population-management-terminology-in-us-health-care.

Penso, J. 2017. "10 Ways to Improve Population Health in 2017." *Becker's Hospital Review*. Published January 9. www.beckershospitalreview.com/population-health/10-ways-to-improve-population-health-in-2017.html.

CHAPTER 7

Reducing Per Capita Cost

INTRODUCTION

As health innovators pursue improved patient experience and population health, the first two anchors of the Triple Aim, they must also pay constant attention to the third: reducing the per capita cost of care. In this chapter, we will explore some of the challenges and opportunities of the shift toward value in healthcare.

Healthcare spending is growing at an unsustainable rate. According to the National Health Expenditure (NHE) Fact Sheet for 2017 (CMS 2018):

- NHE grew 3.9 percent to $3.5 trillion, or $10,739 per person, and accounted for 17.9 percent of gross domestic product (GDP).
- Medicare spending grew 4.2 percent to $705.9 billion, or 20 percent of total NHE.
- Medicaid spending grew 2.9 percent to $589.9 billion, or 17 percent of total NHE.
- Private health insurance spending grew 4.2 percent to $1,183.9 billion, or 34 percent of total NHE.
- Out-of-pocket spending grew 2.6 percent to $365.5 billion, or 10 percent of total NHE.

- Hospital expenditures grew 4.6 percent to $1,142.6 billion, slower than the 5.6 percent growth in 2016.
- Physician and clinical services expenditures grew 4.2 percent to $694.3 billion in 2017, a slower growth than the 5.6 percent in 2016.
- Prescription drug spending increased 0.4 percent to $333.4 billion in 2017, slower than the 2.3 percent growth in 2016.
- The federal government (28.1 percent) and the households (28.0 percent) sponsored the largest shares of total health spending.
- The private business share of health spending accounted for 19.9 percent of total healthcare spending, state and local governments accounted for 17.1 percent, and other private revenues accounted for 6.8 percent (CMS 2018).

The national health spending is projected to grow at an annual average rate of 5.5 percent for 2017–2026 and to reach $5.7 trillion by 2026. While this projected average annual growth rate is more modest than the 7.3 percent observed over the longer-term history

Healthcare Spending

Despite all of the regulation, and a massive new entitlement, [both of which have come about as part of the Affordable Care Act], we have not bent the healthcare cost curve. Healthcare spending is actually growing more quickly now than it was in the year in which the ACA was passed. If we continue on this path, by 2026 we will be spending one in every five dollars on healthcare. Our healthcare system is on an unsustainable trajectory.

—Seema Verma (2018)

(1990–2007), it is more rapid than had been experienced from 2008 to 2016 (4.2 percent). Health spending is projected to grow 1 percent faster than the GDP over the 2017 to 2026 period; as a result, the health share of GDP is expected to rise from 17.9 percent in 2016 to 19.7 percent by 2026 (CMS 2018).

To reduce healthcare costs, the Centers for Medicare & Medicaid Services (CMS) and the Department of Health and Human Services (HHS) focus on implementing value-based purchasing (VBP). This model shifts the healthcare sector away from the traditional fee-for-service model by linking providers' payments to improved performance. It requires providers to demonstrate that they are meeting quality standards and benefiting patients while cutting costs across the continuum of care.

Hospital VBP affects payment for inpatient stays in more than 3,000 hospitals across the country. These hospitals are rewarded (or penalized) based on how well they perform on certain quality measures. A hospital's performance is stacked up against its peers' performance, CMS benchmarks, and its own performance over time.

VALUE-BASED PURCHASING

CMS measures hospital performance on a set of measures and dimensions grouped into specific quality domains with specified weights (percentages). In 2017, the domains and their respective weights included safety (20 percent), clinical care (outcomes 25 percent plus process 5 percent), efficiency and cost reduction (25 percent), and the patient and caregiver-centered experience of care and care coordination (25 percent).

CMS allows hospitals with sufficient data in at least three out of the four domain scores to receive a total performance score (TPS). They earn two scores—one for achievement and another for improvement.

The hospital VBP Program is funded by reducing participating hospitals' Medicare severity diagnosis-related group payments by

2 percent. Any residual funds are redistributed to hospitals based on their TPS.

VBP is not going to fade away, and the shift toward value has only accelerated. In January 2015, the HHS announced its intent to tie 85 percent of all traditional Medicare payments to quality or value by 2016 and to award 90 percent of payments by 2018 through hospital VBP.

CMS also announced several changes to the program for fiscal year 2018. The four domains on which hospitals are now scored—safety, clinical care, efficiency and cost reduction, and patient and caregiver-centered experience of care and care coordination—will be weighted equally at 25 percent each. Beginning with fiscal year 2019, CMS will change the name "patient and caregiver-centered experience of care and care coordination" to "person and community engagement." For 2018, CMS also removed two measures from the clinical care dimension and added a care transition dimension (CMS 2017b).

SHARED SAVINGS

A study in *Internal Medicine* found that accountable care organizations (ACOs) with a strong focus on preventive and postdischarge care benefit from collaboration across care settings, resulting in savings (Colla et al. 2016). Focusing on clinically vulnerable patients—those with serious conditions who are responsible for the greatest proportion of spending—may result in the largest effects on both patient outcomes and financial rewards for participating physician groups. Total spending decreased by $49 per beneficiary-quarter after ACO contract implementation across the overall Medicare population, with a greater decrease of $147 in clinically vulnerable patients.

In the overall Medicare cohort, hospitalizations and emergency department visits decreased by 4.2 and 2.9 events per 1,000 beneficiaries per quarter, and hospitalizations decreased in the clinically vulnerable cohort by 4.9 and 4.1 events per 1000 beneficiaries per quarter. Changes in total spending associated with ACOs did not vary by clinical condition of beneficiaries.

SAFETY NET HOSPITALS

VBP is driving improvements by mandating better care at a lower cost. However, for providers and health systems that cannot achieve the required scores, the financial penalties and lower reimbursements create a significant financial burden.

Safety net hospitals are a category of hospitals that provide a disproportionate level of charity care compared to other facilities. These hospitals receive Disproportionate Share Hospital (DSH) payments from CMS to help offset the cost of caring for large numbers of Medicaid and Medicare beneficiaries, as well as uninsured patients receiving uncompensated care. However, the ACA calls for DSH payments to be significantly reduced over a period of years. DSH funding began in 2014.

Cash-strapped safety net organizations may not have the resources and capital available to completely transition to the VBP system. Safety net organizations are always tight on staff, time, and money, and they struggle to allocate resources to implement innovation effectively. Indeed, the Hospital Readmissions Reduction Program (HRRP) has come under scrutiny for potentially unfairly penalizing safety net systems for factors that contribute to readmissions but that may be beyond their control, such as patients' socioeconomic status or cultural preferences.

One example is Denver Health, a municipal safety net hospital in Colorado, that had an operating income of $5.5 million on patient revenue of $744 million in 2012; in 2011, it posted a net income of $18.3 million. The hospital projected $4.7 million in operating income in its 2013 budget. However, an unexpected increase in the number of uninsured and indigent patients, along with lower reimbursement from Medicare and Medicaid for observation, put the hospital in the red by more than $2 million.

While the ACA alleviated some of these problems by bringing more uninsured patients into the Medicaid system, thus paying the hospital for uncompensated treatment, it is unclear whether the payments it received from Medicaid were sufficient to cover the costs of caring for the newly insured individuals. As a result, the leaders of Denver Health set out to reduce costs by $10 million in 2013 through spending cuts, including staffing and operations (Booth 2013). "Denver Health's challenging payer mix is heavily dependent on governmental sources, safety net reimbursement and supplemental funding, which may be susceptible to funding cuts. However, Denver Health's vital role as the provider of critical public health services to vulnerable populations will ensure that it continues to receive a sufficient level of funding needed to provide these essential services" (Business Wire 2016).

PROPOSED RULE

In April 2017, CMS proposed a rule that included an important modification in how hospitals would be scored (HRRP). The rule, which would take effect in FY 2019, would require Medicare to consider social risk factors when calculating hospital penalties under the HRRP (CMS 2017a).

According to an Advisory Board (Fontana 2017) analysis of the April CMS rule, the federal agency "intends to sort hospitals into five peer groups according to their dual-eligible inpatient stay ratio. Within each peer group, hospitals' excess readmission ratio for each of the program's six conditions will be compared to the groups' median excess readmission ratio for that condition. The proposed change, which is designed to be budget-neutral for Medicare, would shake up the magnitude of HRRP penalties, especially for some safety-net hospitals." This modification was well received by safety net hospitals, which have long felt that HRRP disproportionately and unfairly penalizes them.

Does the HRRP Disproportionately Penalize Safety-Net Hospitals?

A recent *Health Affairs* study finds that persistent penalties under the HRRP could impede hospitals' ability to meet the needs of their communities and invest in quality improvement efforts.

The HRRP aims to reduce costly and preventable hospital readmissions by penalizing hospitals with excess 30-day Medicare readmissions. Despite readmission reductions in response to the program, many experts fear that a disproportionate allocation of penalties ultimately could widen disparities in care.

Researchers found more than half of the hospitals in the study received penalties all five years of the HRRP. Hospitals that were penalized more often in the first years of the program—particularly urban, major teaching, large, and safety net hospitals—were more likely to receive penalties in all five years. The average penalty rose from 0.29 percent in 2013 to 0.60 percent this year. Medium-sized hospitals, as well as hospitals with higher proportions of Medicare patients, saw larger increases in penalties.

Overall, researchers found that hospitals serving a high proportion of socioeconomically disadvantaged patients received more penalties. In addition, safety-net hospitals were not able to improve their readmission rates at the same speed as their non-safety-net counterparts. The researchers recommend developing alternative penalty structures in the HRRP to avoid persistent penalization, while motivating reductions in hospital readmissions.

—Dayna Clark (2017)

KEY TAKEAWAYS

- Under value-based payment, a hospital's performance is compared to that of its peers, CMS benchmarks, and its own past performance.
- Ninety percent of Medicare payments are tied to quality or value.
- Starting in FY 2018, the four domains on which hospitals are scored—safety, clinical care, efficiency and cost reduction, and patient and caregiver-centered experience of care and care coordination—are weighted equally (25 percent each).
- Disproportionate Share Hospital (DSH) payments, under which facilities are able to receive at least partial payments, are expected to decrease over time. However, changes to CMS payment rules may help level the playing field for safety net hospitals.

REFERENCES

Booth, M. 2013. "Denver Health Sinks into Red Again, Cites Cases Others Avoid." *Denver Post*. Published June 24. www.denverpost.com/ci_23524476/denver-health-sinks-into -red-again-cites-cases.

Business Wire. 2016. "Fitch Affirms Denver Health and Hospital Authority (CO) at 'BBB+'; Outlook Stable." Published May 13. www.businesswire.com/news/home/20160513005728/en/ Fitch-Affirms-Denver-Health-Hospital-Authority-BBB.

Centers for Medicare & Medicaid Services (CMS). 2018. "NHE Fact Sheet." Modified December 6. www.cms.gov/research -statistics-data-and-systems/statistics-trends-and-reports/ nationalhealthexpenddata/nhe-fact-sheet.html.

————. 2017a. "Fiscal Year (FY) 2018 Medicare Hospital Inpatient Prospective Payment System (IPPS) and Long Term Acute Care Hospital (LTCH) Prospective Payment System Proposed Rule, and Request for Information CMS-1677-P." Published April 14. www.cms.gov/newsroom/fact-sheets/fiscal-year-fy -2018-medicare-hospital-inpatient-prospective-payment-system -ipps-and-long-term-acute.

————. 2017b. *Hospital Value-Based Purchasing*. Published September. www.cms.gov/Outreach-and-Education/Medi- care-Learning-Network-MLN/MLNProducts/downloads/ Hospital_VBPurchasing_Fact_Sheet_ICN907664.pdf.

Clark, D. 2017. "Study: HRRP Disproportionately Penalizes Safety- Net Hospitals." America's Essential Hospitals. Published July 13. https://essentialhospitals.org/institute/safety-net-hospitals -disproportionately-penalized-under-hospital-readmissions -reduction-program-hrrp/.

Colla, C. H., V. A. Lewis, L. Kao, A. J. O'Malley, C. Chang, and E. S. Fisher. 2016. "Association Between Medicare Account- able Care Organization Implementation and Spending Among Clinically Vulnerable Beneficiaries." *JAMA Internal Medicine* 176 (8): 1167–75

Fontana, E. 2017. "Early Impressions: CMS's FY 2018 Inpa- tient Proposed Rule." Advisory Board. Published April 17. www.advisory.com/research/financial-leadership-council/ at-the-margins/2017/04/ipps-rule.

Verma, S. 2018. "Speech: Remarks by CMS Administrator Seema Verma at the American Hospital Association Annual Mem- bership Meeting." Centers for Medicare & Medicaid Services. Published May 7. www.cms.gov/newsroom/fact-sheets/speech -remarks-cms-administrator-seema-verma-american-hospital -association-annual-membership-meeting.

CHAPTER 8

Accountable Care Organization Models

INTRODUCTION

Accountable care organizations (ACOs) facilitate coordination and cooperation among groups of primary care physicians, specialists, and post-acute providers. These caregivers must have a minimum of 5,000 Medicare beneficiaries, and they take joint responsibility in providing high-quality care to the Medicare patients they serve. ACOs ensure that patients, especially the chronically ill, receive the right care at the right time, with the goal of avoiding unnecessary duplication of services and preventing medical errors (CMS 2019).

ACOs are designed to overcome the inconsistent and unco-ordinated care delivered by independent primary care physicians and hospitals. They are also an attempt to overcome the pitfalls of the fee-for-service (FFS) payment system, which rewards providers for the number of services they provide rather than the quality or value of those services. The strategic intent of such organizations is the simultaneous pursuit of the Triple Aim: improving the patient experience of care (including quality and satisfaction), improving the health of populations, and reducing the per capita cost of health-care. This chapter addresses structural and regulatory requirements associated with the formation of ACOs, risk factors and financial incentives, performance outcomes, and revisions to the current ACO participation models.

ACCOUNTABLE CARE ORGANIZATION OUTCOMES

By August 2017, there were 428 Medicare Shared Savings Program (MSSP) ACOs serving 9.7 million beneficiaries. A year later, in August 2018, the number jumped to 561 participating ACOs serving more than 10.5 million Medicare FFS beneficiaries (CMS 2018b).

From 2013 to 2016, the Medicare ACOs collectively achieved a net spending reduction of nearly $1 billion while improving the quality of care delivery on most (82 percent) of the individual quality measures. The Office of Inspector General of the Department of Health and Human Services also indicated that over the first three years of the program, ACOs outperformed FFS providers on most (81 percent) of the quality measures. Further, a small subset of high-performing ACOs reduced spending by an average of $673 per beneficiary for key Medicare services during that period. In contrast, other MSSP ACOs and the national average for FFS providers showed an increase in per beneficiary spending for key Medicare services (US Department of Health and Human Services 2017).

MEDICARE ACCESS AND CHIP REAUTHORIZATION ACT OF 2015

The Medicare Access and CHIP Reauthorization Act of 2015 (MACRA) was signed into law on April 16, 2015. It is a method for ensuring that the yearly increase in the expense per Medicare beneficiary will not exceed the growth in gross domestic product.

Every year, the Centers for Medicare & Medicaid Services (CMS) sends a report to the Medicare Payment Advisory Commission, which advises Congress on the previous year's total expenditures and the target expenditures. The report also includes a conversion factor that would change the payments for physician services for the next year in order to match the target sustainable growth rate (SGR).

On March 1 of each year, if the expenditures for the previous year exceed the target expenditures, then the conversion factor would decrease payments for the subsequent year. If the expenditures for the previous year were less than expected, the conversion factor would increase the payments to physicians in subsequent years. MACRA created the Quality Payment Program, which effectively:

- Replaced the previous SGR method.
- Changed the way that Medicare rewards providers for value over volume.
- Streamlined existing quality programs (i.e., Physician Quality Reporting Program [PQRS], Value Based Payment Modifier [VBM]) that measure the quality and cost of care provided to people with Medicare under the Medicare Physician Fee Schedule, the electronic health record (EHR) Incentive Program, and meaningful use (MU), with a focus on interoperability and information exchange. These programs are clustered under the new Merit-based Incentive Payments System (MIPS) with the requirement to report improvement activities on an annual basis.
- Provided bonus payments for participation in eligible alternative payment models (APMs) that treat similar care episodes and clinical condition groups across settings (CMS 2018d).

Scores in the four performance categories are weighted and rolled up into the MIPS final score (0–100) and are compared against a threshold (see exhibit 8.1). The final score determines the clinician's payment adjustments (American Academy of Family Physicians 2019). Absence of an EHR offsets the weighted points under that performance category. Qualified physicians participating in MIPS in 2018 will be eligible for positive or negative Medicare Part B payment adjustments of up to 5 percent.

Exhibit 8.1: Merit-Based Incentive Payments System

Performance Category	2018 (%)	2019 (%)	2020 (%)
Quality (PQRS/VBM)	50	30	30
Cost (resource utilization)	10	30	30
Interoperability (EHR/MU)	25	25	25
Improvement activities	15	15	15

Note: PQRS = Physician Quality Reporting Program, VBM = Value Based Payment Modifier, EHR = electronic health record, MU = meaningful use.

BUNDLED PAYMENTS AND RISK STRATIFICATION

ACOs use a bundled payment model that focuses on coordinated, value-based care that aligns incentives with measurable quality, cost reduction and operational efficiency, and improved population health outcomes. The alternative payment model also encourages providers to gather data from across the continuum of care to identify cost-effective care pathways for episodes. Under a bundled payment model, the payer would reimburse providers and healthcare facilities for episode-based services within a defined period using a set price.

Successful ACOs are able to decrease overall healthcare costs, eliminate unnecessary duplication of services, and reduce medical errors. ACOs that exceed the benchmarked reimbursement for the episode are responsible for the financial burden of overages. When the cost of the episode is less than the bundled payment price, providers keep the savings. However, if the cost exceeds the set price, participating parties bear the difference.

In some cases, payers reimburse one of the entities involved in the care delivery process and that party, in turn, apportions the payment among the providers. In others, payers reimburse each participating provider separately, while ensuring that the aggregate payment does not exceed the set price.

One of the major challenges of bundled payments is managing costs for a patient's treatment that may be out of the provider's control—for example, adverse events resulting from nonadherence. Other challenges include fixed costs and high overhead, which may limit providers' financial ability to sustain an income reduction (should treatment costs exceed the set price); insufficient funding for implementing EHR and data system interoperability; and cost overrun resulting from intensive case management for high-risk patients.

HIERARCHICAL CONDITION CATEGORY

CMS designed a Hierarchical Condition Category (HCC) risk-adjustment model to calculate risk scores. The CMS-HCC risk-adjustment model is prospective: it uses health status in a base year to predict costs in the subsequent year. Higher categories with higher predicted healthcare costs, such as long-term chronic obstructive pulmonary disease (COPD), chronic heart failure (CHF), and diabetes are given higher risk scores. Acute illnesses and injuries, however, are not reliably predictive of ongoing healthcare costs. For a diagnosis to factor into risk adjustment, it must be evidence based (derived from medical records and provider–patient encounters), documented at least once per year, and coded according to the ICD-10-CM guidelines (Centers for Disease Control and Prevention 2019).

According to physician-scholars J. Michael McWilliams and Aaron L. Schwartz (2017), focusing on patients with high spending may not necessarily target the spending that should be reduced, because patients' needs fluctuate randomly, sometimes as a result of risk factors that are not clearly apparent or cannot be measured. "We found that 75 percent of Medicare spending was concentrated among 17 percent of beneficiaries in 2013, but high-risk patients identified by means of predictive information accounted for a smaller proportion of spending. For example, care for the 17 percent of Medicare beneficiaries with the highest HCC risk scores and most chronic conditions in 2013 cost nearly four times as much per person as care for other beneficiaries but accounted for only 42 percent of Medicare spending." McWilliams and Schwartz concluded, "Patient-focused strategies applied to high-risk patients must be substantially more effective or less costly than broader strategies to justify their prominence in cost-containment efforts."

Providers may also want to identify alternative risk stratification methods that consider different categories based on patients' use of services and calculate a risk score to predict patients' needs throughout the episode of care, especially if it falls under the set price of the bundled payment. Risk stratification enables providers to better understand their patient populations, manage their resources more effectively, train staff for transitional care, and develop action planning for inpatient and outpatient settings. Lindsey Haas and colleagues (2013) of the Mayo Clinic's Employee and Community Health practice (a primary care division of the Minnesota group) compared different risk-stratification methods to determine which best predicts outcomes in subsequent years.

The researchers used retrospective cohort analysis to identify high-risk patients among more than 83,000 patient records from 2009 to 2010, prior to the start of care coordination in 2011. Adjusted clinical groups (ACGs), a population and patient-case-mix adjustment system developed by the School of Public Health at Johns Hopkins University that clusters clients into homogenous groups, have been found to improve accuracy and fairness in forecasting healthcare utilization. They also predict inpatient hospitalizations as well as, or better than, other case-mix models in many health systems. The study concluded that the use of any of these models would help health providers implement care coordination more efficiently.

ACCOUNTABLE CARE ORGANIZATION MODELS

Bundled payments shift financial and clinical accountability to the ACO, which is responsible for the resources and quality of care delivered for any given episode. The ACO earns a higher margin with low-risk patients but also bears the financial risk of (re)admissions and complications for high-risk patients.

This payment model incentivizes coordinated care across settings. Payers and providers can choose an upside track or prospective payment model (track 1 before services are rendered) or a downside track or retrospective two-sided model (tracks 2 and 3 after all services are rendered).

Track 1, a one-sided shared savings track, allows ACOs to receive additional reimbursement of up to 50 percent of savings under the benchmark without assuming any responsibility for potential losses should spending exceed the benchmark. ACOs can remain in track 1 for up to six years transitioning to a two-sided model. As exhibit 8.2 shows, the vast majority of MSSP ACOs (82 percent) participate in track 1.

ACOs participating in tracks 2 and 3, the two-sided model with shared savings and shared losses, are eligible to receive a larger portion of any savings. However, they are also required to endure downside risks, repaying shared losses to CMS if their spending exceeds the benchmark. Participation in track 2 has decreased over the years (to only eight ACOs), especially after the 2016 introduction of track 3, the program's highest-risk track (which also has the highest level of potential reward). Track 3 currently has 38 participants. The track 1+ model, introduced in January 2018 to accelerate the progress of track 1 ACOs undertaking performance-based risk, is a two-sided model with a lower downside; 55 ACOs are members. As of January 2018, physician-only ACOs accounted for 30 percent, or 171, of the 561 ACOs in the MSSP (see exhibit 8.2).

Avalere's analysis of the downside-risk models in the MSSP (tracks 2 and 3) has shown significant savings to the Medicare program and improved quality. As the number of downside-risk ACOs increases over time, the model has the potential for creating greater savings for CMS. During 2012–2017, the upside-only model (MSSP track 1) increased federal spending by $444 million compared to the downside-risk ACOs that reduced federal spending by $60 million (Seidman, Feore, and Rosacker 2018).

Exhibit 8.2: ACO Models: Participation and Performance

Medicare Shared Savings Program
Fast Facts

HISTORICAL PARTICIPATION AND PERFORMANCE

PROGRAM CHARACTERISTICS

Performance Year	ACOs	Assigned Beneficiaries
2018	561	10.5 million
2017	480	9.0 million
2016	433	7.7 million
2015	404	7.3 million
2014	338	4.9 million
2012/2013	220	3.2 million

PERFORMANCE YEAR RESULTS

Performance Year 2016
Total Earned Performance Payments	$700,607,912
Average Overall Quality Score	94.65%

Performance Year 2015
Total Earned Performance Payments	$645,543,866
Average Overall Quality Score	91.44%

Performance Year 2014
Total Earned Performance Payments	$341,246,303
Average Overall Quality Score	83.08%

Performance Year 2012/13
Total Earned Performance Payments	$315,908,772
Average Overall Quality Score	95.00%

ACO PARTICIPANT LIST COMPOSITION

Participant TINs	20,690
Physicians, PAs, NPs, CNSs	377,515
Hospitals	1,517
Federally Qualified Health Centers	2,560
Rural Health Centers	1,210
Critical Access Hospitals	421

SNF AFFILIATES (SNF 3-DAY RULE WAIVER)

SNFs	868

2018 ACCOUNTABLE CARE ORGANIZATION INFORMATION

ACO CHARACTERISTICS

	ACOs	Percent
Non-Risk Based:		
Track 1	460	82%
Risk Based:		
Track 1+ Model	55	10%
SNF 3-Day Rule Waiver	31	–
Track 2	8	1%
Track 3	38	7%
SNF 3-Day Rule Waiver	30	–

ACO COMPOSITION

	ACOs	Percent
Physicians Only	171	30%
Physicians, Hospitals, & Other Facilities	324	58%
FQHCs/RHCs	66	12%

2018 MEDICARE BENEFICIARY DEMOGRAPHIC DISTRIBUTION

	Beneficiary Person-Years	Percent
ESRD	81,397	0.79%
Disabled	1,294,555	12.64%
Aged Dual	688,076	6.72%
Aged Non-Dual	8,180,954	79.85%

Source: Reprinted from CMS (2018b).

REVAMPING THE ACCOUNTABLE CARE ORGANIZATION MODELS

On August 9, 2018, CMS issued a proposed rule that would accelerate the shift to two-sided risk (in which the organization may share in savings and is accountable for repaying shared losses) while promoting competition by encouraging participation in the model by low-revenue ACOs. Referred to as "Pathways to Success," or "glide paths," this proposed rule for the MSSP would encourage ACOs to transition to two-sided models. According to CMS, the program changes "are designed to increase savings for the Trust Funds (which finance health services for beneficiaries of Medicare) and mitigate losses, reduce gaming opportunities (e.g., cost-shifting), and promote regulatory flexibility and free-market principles." The transition to two-sided risk models is projected to increase program integrity, enhance the use of interoperable EHRs among ACO providers and suppliers, and promote healthy competition in the marketplace (CMS 2018c).

ACOs with a participation agreement ending on December 31, 2018, have the option to extend their current agreement period for an additional six-month performance year and may apply for a new agreement beginning on July 1, 2019. This would provide ACOs sufficient time to review new policies, make business and investment decisions, obtain a buy-in from their governing bodies and executives, and complete and submit an application for the MSSP beginning July 1, 2019. CMS would resume the full annual application cycle for the performance year on January 1, 2020.

Starting July 1, 2019, eligible ACOs would enter an agreement period of at least five years through two options: (1) a BASIC track, which has the same maximum level of risk as track 1+, and (2) the ENHANCED track, based on the program's existing track 3. CMS will also provide additional tools and flexibility for ACOs that take on the highest level of risk and potential reward. The proposed rule changes the low-risk participation limit from six years to two years

Cleveland Clinic's Medicare ACO Transitions to Track 1+ Advanced Payment Model

Under the new model, Cleveland Clinic Medicare ACO, which manages a population of 105,000 beneficiaries, will assume limited performance-based downside risk if it doesn't meet a savings threshold, in addition to the opportunity to share in savings based on its quality performance.

With the downside risk of a fixed 30 percent loss sharing rate comes the potential for rewards in terms of shared savings (up to 50 percent). The new model, called track 1+, qualifies Cleveland Clinic Medicare ACO as an Advanced Payment Model under the Medicare Access and CHIP Reauthorization Act of 2015 (MACRA), allowing all its participant providers to meet MACRA's quality reporting requirements and provide the health system with greater Medicare reimbursement for physician services starting in 2019.

Through Cleveland Clinic Community Health, a new population management-focused initiative, Cleveland Clinic is well positioned to manage its Medicare population efficiently and holistically and, by leveraging more robust analytics on beneficiaries, can assume greater risk.

Under Track 1+, Cleveland Clinic Medicare ACO will have prospective beneficiary assignment that allows it to know in advance the patient population for which it is responsible, and the option to request a Skilled Nursing Facility 3-Day Rule Waiver to provide greater flexibility to better coordinate and deliver high-quality care.

In 2016, the ACO had $42.2 million in savings, which was a 24.5 percent increase from 2015. Also in 2016, it received $19.9 million back in shared savings, a 19.8 percent increase over 2015, and the health system's quality score was 96.3 percent.

—Cleveland Clinic (2018)

for first-time ACOs and to one year for returning ACOs. Tracks 1 and 2 will eventually be phased out.

The BASIC track includes five levels: a one-sided model available only for the first two years to eligible ACOs (previous track 1 participants), and three levels of progressively higher risk and potential reward in years 3–5 of the agreement period. Under the one-sided model years of the glide path, an ACO's maximum shared-savings rate would be 25 percent, with a cap of 50 percent, based on the quality performance sharing rate and a maximum level of risk that qualifies as an advanced APM.

On December 21, 2018, CMS published its final rule, which included two big changes to what it initially recommended in the proposed rule. CMS agreed to provide some flexibility by allowing new, nonreentering, low-revenue ACOs (many of which are in rural areas) up to three years under the one-sided model. CMS also finalized a higher initial shared savings rate, up from 25 percent to 40 percent for one-sided risk ACOs. The shared savings rate for ACOs at all levels of risk will remain at 50 percent under this final rule. ACOs in the BASIC-track glide path would be automatically progressing at the start of each performance year, along the levels of risk and reward, or they could elect to accelerate their progression to higher levels of risk and reward over the course of their agreement period.

While the typical agreement period under the proposed rule would be five years, with twelve-month performance years based on calendar years, ACOs entering an agreement period beginning on July 1, 2019, would participate in a first performance year of six months for the period July–December 2019. ACOs entering the BASIC track's glide path for an agreement period beginning on July 1, 2019, would have at most two and a half years under a one-sided model (with ACOs identified as having previously participated in the program under track 1 restricted to one and a half years), with their first automatic advancement starting in 2021.

ACOs less experienced with performance-based Medicare ACO initiatives may enter an agreement period under the BASIC track's glide path. More experienced ACOs (e.g., those that have previously participated in tracks 2 or 3, or even track 1+) are restricted to participating in either the BASIC track's highest level of risk and reward or the ENHANCED track. ACOs identified as low revenue could participate in the BASIC track for up to two agreement periods. They also have the option to renew under the BASIC track, at the highest level of risk and reward, for a second agreement period. ACOs identified as high revenue would be required to transition to the ENHANCED track more quickly, after no more than a single agreement period under the BASIC track (CMS 2018c).

ESTIMATED IMPACT

CMS estimates that the proposed changes will save Medicare $2.24 billion from 2019 to 2028 while simultaneously improving interoperability and coordination of care. The trade-offs, however, include the projection that by 2028, 109 fewer ACOs would participate in the MSSP (see exhibit 8.3).

The National Association of ACOs (NAACOS 2018) conducted a survey of the 82 ACOs that began the MSSP in 2012 or 2013 and remained in track 1 (the upside track) in 2018. The objective was to get a sense of their future participation plans in the required two-sided ACO model and assess how they felt about risk. The majority of the respondents (71.4 percent) indicated they are likely to leave the MSSP, citing the following reasons:

- The amount of risk was too great (39.4 percent).
- Unpredictable changes to the ACO model and CMS rules (39.4 percent).
- Desire for more reliable financial projections (39.4 percent).

Clif Gaus, NAACOS president and CEO, projected that "many ACOs (will) quit the program, divest their care coordination resources and return to payment models that emphasize volume over value. This would be a real setback for Medicare payment reform efforts" (NAACOS 2018). One of the main concerns is that many ACOs will be left with a single year to collect relevant performance data prior to evaluating the required transition to risk in their third year of the program. Nevertheless, in its final rule from December 21, 2018, CMS responded partially but effectively to some of the criticisms by modifying the shared savings rates, rewarding participating ACOs that take on greater risk with higher shared-savings rates.

Exhibit 8.3 summarizes the annual projected mean impact of the proposed changes on ACO participation, federal spending on Medicare Parts A and B claims, ACO earnings from the shared savings net of shared losses, and the net federal impact (the effect on claims, net of the change in shared savings and in shared losses payments). The overall average projection of the impact of the proposed program changes is approximately $2.24 billion in lower overall federal spending over ten years. Impact on claims, ACO shared savings, advanced APM incentive payments, and net federal spending are expressed in millions of dollars.

The overall drop in expected participation is attributed to the shift from six years in track 1 to two years in the BASIC track, which is also less attractive with its lower 25 percent maximum sharing rate during the two risk-free years. Nonetheless, CMS predicts that the changes are expected to increase participation from existing ACOs. These included organizations currently facing mandated transition to risk in a third agreement period starting in 2019, 2020, or 2021 under the existing regulations, as well as higher-cost ACOs for whom the capped regional adjustment would not reduce their benchmark as significantly as prescribed by current regulation (CMS 2018a).

Exhibit 8.3: Ten-Year Estimated Impact of Proposed Rule

Performance Year	ACO Participation	Claims	ACO Net Earnings	Federal Impact Before APM Incentives	Advanced APM Incentives to QPs	Net Federal Impact
2019	−20	60	60	120	0	120
2020	−33	80	40	120	0	120
2021	−49	50	20	70	0	70
2022	−29	20	−150	−130	70	−60
2023	−17	−40	−200	−240	130	−110
2024	−21	−110	−160	−280	220	−60
2025	−90	−160	−290	−450	0	−450
2026	−109	−190	−400	−590	30	−560
2027	−107	−150	−500	−650	0	−650
2028	−109	−80	−570	−650	−10	−660
10-Year Total		**−510**	**−2,170**	**−2,680**	**440**	**−2,240**
Low (10th Percentile)		−2,140	−4,310	−4,840	110	−4,430
High (90th Percentile)		1,040	−270	−440	740	90

Source: Reprinted from CMS (2018a).

PHYSICIAN-LED ACCOUNTABLE CARE ORGANIZATIONS

Researchers have found that the longer physician-led ACOs participated in the MSSP, the more significant the savings (McWilliams et al. 2018). By 2015, physician-led ACOs participating in the CMS Pioneer Model (ACOs that entered the program in 2012) yielded $474 in savings per Medicare beneficiary, compared to $342 for those entering in 2013 and $156 for those entering in 2014.

To compare, hospital-led ACOs that entered the program in 2012 only saw $169 in savings per Medicare beneficiary, which declined to $18 for the 2013 group and $88 for those entering in 2014. While spending reductions in physician-led ACOs led to $256.4 million in net savings in 2015, spending reductions in hospital-led ACOs were offset by bonus payments, costing the program money.

By January 2018, physician-only ACOs accounted for 30 percent (171) of the 561 MSSP ACOs (see exhibit 8.2). Participating in physician-led ACOs appears to be an attractive alternative to consolidation with larger hospitals or health systems, allowing physicians to provide high-quality care at a reasonable price while retaining their independence (Lemaire and Singer 2018). Some physician-only ACOs implemented EHR software and established care coordination and compliance infrastructure. They did so by working with third-party vendors who accepted contingency payments based on future savings (Matsakis 2018). A physician-led ACO gives physicians the opportunity to engage in senior governance roles in addition to shaping the quality and cost of care delivery.

Waivers of the Stark Act and the Anti-Kickback Statute provide MSSP ACOs and their participants with broad protection against fraud and abuse prosecution if all requirements are met. The waivers also open the door for physician leaders to engage innovatively and collaboratively with unaffiliated practices and hospitals.

REDUCING THE RISK

ACOs are not limited to collaborating only with regional groups of health providers. As with most business ventures, spreading out the risk over more partners may be safer. Covering a large number of beneficiaries may also spread the risk of fixed costs. Strategies to reduce unnecessary costs or variances and driving lower-cost utilization should not focus solely on intensive case management for high-cost patients but on services that are of low value (McWilliams et al. 2018). Reinvesting a portion of the global payment fee to support the ACO capabilities and engage in meaningful collaborative efforts with community public health agencies can also help to improve existing partnerships and coordinated care (Lewis et al. 2014).

Creative dyad leaders may employ the establishment of an ACO as an opportunity to organize a common purpose while permitting the individual partners to retain some measure of cultural distinction.

Palm Beach ACO Doctors Top Nation in Medicare Savings

A doctor group based in Palm Beach County leads the country in saving taxpayers money while meeting goals for keeping Medicare patients happy and healthy.

Palm Beach Accountable Care Organization based in Palm Springs saved taxpayers $62 million and was allowed to keep $30 million of that for 2016 because it earned high scores for patient health and satisfaction, according to federal officials. The group ranked No. 2 nationally in shared savings a year ago.

"We're keeping our patients healthier and out of the hospital," said board chairperson Richard Weisberg. "The savings are good and we're proud of those. Keeping patients healthy is most important."

The group of 275 primary-care doctors and 175 specialists serves 69,000 Medicare patients from St. Lucie County to Miami-Dade County.

—Charles Elmore (2018)

According to public health scholars Karen Hacker and Deborah Klein Walker (2013), an ACO's integrated strategy should be committed to serving the health of the people in the communities from which their population is drawn—not just the population of patients enrolled in their care. Strategies they proposed are still relevant and worth careful exploration. Consider the following:

- Determining the regional communities in which patients reside and the overlap between the ACO and the community population.

- Comparing the health of the population served by the ACO with that of the community.
- Deciding what level of overlap in any geographic area merits collaboration. The more market share an ACO has, the more investment in collaboration might be made and the more impact that investment will have on health outcomes.
- Partnering with public health and key community agencies to conduct a joint needs assessment and collaboratively select health outcomes for focus.
- Setting up a formal agreement with the public health authorities to share data and monitor progress toward goals in clinical and community settings.
- Identifying population health indicators to be included on the ACO dashboard.

KEY TAKEAWAYS

- Bundled payments maximize value for the patient because payments cover the overall care and are linked to important outcomes.
- Bundled payments create incentives for clinical integration and joint accountability in which clinical teams are empowered to add services not covered by a FFS set-up but that add value for patients.
- Physician-led ACOs typically outperform hospital-led ACOs, improving quality and producing greater savings.
- ACOs that take on greater levels of risk achieve better results than ACOs that select one-sided risk.
- CMS will continue to pressure providers to assume greater risks and to provide evidence of quality care and safety.
- Clinical integration, interoperability, and risk sharing among providers will continue to dominate the healthcare field.

- CMS encourages private insurers and large employers to adopt APMs.
- APMs are "patient friendly," as they incentivize high quality, cost-effective, coordinated care with a focus on better patient outcomes.

REFERENCES

American Academy of Family Physicians. 2019. "Frequently Asked Questions: Medicare Access and CHIP Reauthorization Act of 2015 (MACRA)." Published February. www.aafp.org/practice -management/payment/medicare-payment/macra-101/faq .html.

Centers for Disease Control and Prevention. 2019. "ICD-10-CM Official Guidelines for Coding and Reporting." Accessed February 21. www.cdc.gov/nchs/data/icd/10cmguidelines_fy2018_ final.pdf.

Centers for Medicare & Medicaid Services (CMS). 2019. "Accountable Care Organizations (ACOs): General Information." Updated February 15. https://innovation.cms.gov/initiatives/aco.

————. 2018a. "Medicare Program; Medicare Shared Savings Program; Accountable Care Organizations—Pathways to Success." Published August 17. https://s3.amazonaws.com/public-inspection.federalregister.gov/2018-17101.pdf.

————. 2018b. "Medicare Shared Savings Program Fast Facts." Published January. www.cms.gov/Medicare/Medicare-Fee -for-Service-Payment/sharedsavingsprogram/Downloads/ SSP-2018-Fast-Facts.pdf.

————. 2018c. "Proposed Pathways to Success for the Medicare Shared Savings Program." Published August 9. www.cms.gov/ newsroom/fact-sheets/proposed-pathways-success-medicare -shared-savings-program.

————. 2018d. "What's MACRA?" Modified September 21. www. cms.gov/Medicare/Quality-Initiatives-Patient-Assessment -Instruments/Value-Based-Programs/MACRA-MIPS-and -APMs/MACRA-MIPS-and-APMs.html.

Cleveland Clinic. 2018. "Cleveland Clinic's Medicare Accountable Care Organization (ACO) Transitions to a New Payment Model." Published February 1. https://newsroom.clevelandclinic .org/2018/02/01/cleveland-clinics-medicare-accountable-care -organization-aco-transitions-to-new-advanced-payment-model.

Elmore, C. 2018. "Palm Beach ACO Doctors Top Nation in Medi- care Savings." *Palm Beach Post.* Published May 23. http:// protectingyourpocket.blog.palmbeachpost.com/2017/11/14/ palm-beach-aco-doctors-top-nation-in-medicare-savings/.

Haas, L. R., P. Y. Takahashi, N. D. Shah, R. J. Stroebel, M. E. Ber- nard, D. M. Finnie, and J. M. Naessens. 2013. "Risk-Stratifica- tion Methods for Identifying Patients for Care Coordination." *American Journal of Managed Care* 19 (9): 725–32.

Hacker, K., and D. K. Walker. 2013. "Achieving Population Health in Accountable Care Organizations." *American Journal of Public Health* 103 (7): 1163–67.

Lemaire, N., and S. J. Singer. 2018. "Do Independent Physician-Led ACOs Have a Future?" Published February 22. https://catalyst .nejm.org/do-independent-physician-led-acos-have-a-future.

Lewis, V. A., C. H. Colla, K. E. Schoenherr, S. M. Shortell, and E. S. Fisher. 2014. "Innovation in the Safety Net: Integrating Community Health Centers Through Accountable Care." *Journal of General Internal Medicine* 29 (11): 1484–90.

Matsakis, E. N. 2018. "Physician Only ACOs: An Opportunity to Consider." Accessed February 21. www.ama-assn.org/sites/ default/files/media-browser/public/government/advocacy/ physician-aco.pdf.

McWilliams, J. M., L. A. Hatfield, B. E. Landon, and P. Hamed. 2018. "Medicare Spending After 3 Years of the Medicare Shared

Savings Program." *New England Journal of Medicine* 379 (12): 1139–49.

McWilliams, J. M., and A. L. Schwartz. 2017. "Focusing on High-Cost Patients: The Key to Addressing High Costs?" *New England Journal of Medicine* 376 (9): 807–9.

National Association of ACOs (NAACOS). 2018. "Press Release." Published May 2. www.naacos.com/press-release-may-2-2018.

Seidman, J., J. Feore, and N. Rosacker. 2018. "Medicare Accountable Care Organizations Have Increased Federal Spending Contrary to Projections That They Would Produce Net Savings." Avalere. Published March 29. http://avalere.com/expertise/managed-care/insights/medicare-accountable-care-organizations-have-increased-federal-spending-contrary-to-projections-that-they-would-produce-net-savings.

US Department of Health and Human Services. 2017. "Medicare Shared Savings Program Accountable Care Organizations Have Shown Potential for Reducing Spending and Improving Quality." Published August 28. https://oig.hhs.gov/oei/reports/oei-02-15-00450.asp.

CHAPTER 9

Innovation and Culture

INTRODUCTION

Shaping culture is one of the most important responsibilities of dyad leaders. Building and sustaining adaptive culture is essential for the success of clinical integration (CI).

Achieving an accountable care organization–integrated strategy requires the pursuit of external partnerships, clinical integration, and realignment of organizational processes along the lines of safety and reliability. Culture supports the implementation of strategic initiatives and strategy reinforces elements of a strong adaptive culture.

Creating a culture of interprofessional collaboration and cross-functional synergies reinforces the execution of the accountable care organization (ACO) strategy. The framework explored in this chapter will allow you to conduct a cultural mapping of your health system.

Four types of cultures are described in this chapter: innovation, performance, efficiency, and collaboration. You will be able to use the model described in this chapter to identify underlying values and beliefs held by members about how well the hospital adapts to the changing conditions of the healthcare environment.

CULTURAL TYPES

Four types of purposeful cultures are shown in exhibit 9.1. These four types of cultures are consistent with the dimensions and quadrants of the frameworks discussed earlier in the book (see chapter 3). These cultural types help dyad leaders to diagnose and analyze how well their leadership roles align with or reflect the interests and goals of the health system.

Dyad leaders create opportunities for transformations in a culture of change and innovation and the alignment with the goals of the community. They also sense the need to maintain stability, predictability, and order through a culture of efficiency. They drive value

Exhibit 9.1: Types of Cultures

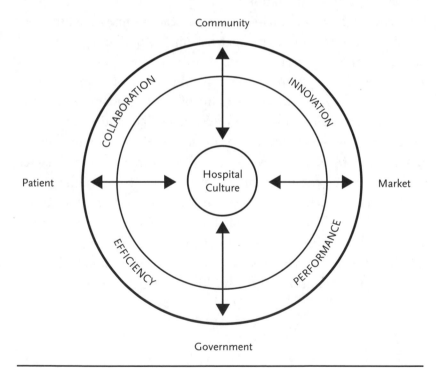

through strategic positioning, economies of scale, and a culture of performance and competition. They focus on culture of collaboration, teamwork, and interprofessional cooperation by promoting transparency, honesty, and trust.

The cultural type of innovation corresponds to the dyad innovator role; performance culture fits with the role of the value strategist; the culture of efficiency matches the role of the CI champion; and the culture that focuses on collaboration reflects characteristics essential for the success of the dyad in the patient advocate role. The following sections discuss dynamics of change and resistance that dyad leaders can expect in each type (Plsek 2014).

Innovation Culture

An *innovation* culture reflects a dynamic, entrepreneurial, and creative health system. Members are risk takers. Leadership is visionary, innovative, and risk oriented. Commitment to innovation is the value that holds members and partners together. The dyad supports clinicians and personnel who initiate new ideas to realign clinical processes with reasonable precautions to avoid harm to patients or the organization.

Innovation is viewed as a deliberate process. The hospital supports formal training about innovation and encourages members of staff to develop their skills and expertise in areas such as problem-solving, brainstorming, and creative thinking. Potential obstacles may include an inadequate number of advocates and sponsors resulting from lack of experience or competency in innovation. Methods and approaches that are quite restrictive hold back the creative process.

Mitigating resistance is critical. Partners who fear reporting errors or perceive that they will appear unwise or lose credibility may resist innovation or become risk averse. Innovation occurs incrementally or progressively by tweaking existing processes, rather than by reframing existing structures through fundamental redesign.

Performance Culture

A performance culture is characterized by a focus on the external environment and on managing transactions with external constituencies, including payers, partners, and regulators. The organization is a results-oriented workplace. Leaders are hard-driving producers and competitors. Value is placed on competitive actions and on meeting goals and targets.

Dyad leaders support change champions and innovators with the funding, time, authority, and empowerment to devote their attention to the process of innovation. Some resistance may occur, too. Because the market culture emphasizes high performance, innovation is viewed as an add-on responsibility to people's regular jobs, potentially reducing their focus and energy for innovation. Financial resources and analytics may also be inadequate (i.e., data of insufficient quantity or type) to support experimentation and testing. In these areas, the role of middle managers in innovation implementation is critical in planning and facilitating execution plans (Belasen and Belasen 2016).

Efficiency Culture

An efficiency culture is characterized by a structured and disciplined workplace. Rules and procedures govern members' actions. Leaders are good coordinators and monitors who help to maintain efficient operations. Value is placed on stability, predictability, optimizing resource use, analytics, and operating efficiency. Information that might help stimulate new thinking is obtained from a variety of sources, both inside and outside the organization.

Information is shared freely and rapidly, without filters or censors, to help foster innovation. Communication is clear and teamwork is trustworthy. Team members are diverse and approach the issue jointly, though from different perspectives. People honor ideas from each other and from nontraditional sources. There is mutual respect and honesty in teams.

Potential barriers may include limited transfer of knowledge and insufficient sharing of best practices across specialized lines that are bound by discipline. Information may be shared on a need-to-know basis only. Benchmarking activities are not supported because of a belief that "we know everything" or "we are different, and it won't work here."

To reduce disagreements, teams are homogeneous, adhering to specialized knowledge and possessing similar skills, experiences, and points of view. Interfunctional collaboration, of course, alters the fabric of these interactions, behaviors, and outcomes.

Collaboration Culture

The collaboration culture is supportive and interactive, as if it were an extended family. Leaders are mentors and coaches. Individual development, high cohesion, morale, teamwork, and consensus are valued. Success is defined in terms of trust, mutual respect, and engagement.

Individuals, as well as groups, are recognized and praised for taking calculated risks, innovating thinking, and championing change. Recognition is individualized to match what the member considers a reward, such as additional time for innovation, peer recognition, or access to decision-making centers in the organization. The innovation activity is energizing, satisfying, and challenging, and thereby intrinsically motivating to participants. Potential barriers to change may include the perception of innovation as a punishing process, as it might be viewed as outside the comfort zone of team members or as a result of insufficient resources. For example, protected time to innovate is not provided, and the process is perceived as a burden. Innovation is not well integrated in the performance review process. Ideas that are not executed well are ridiculed, rather than being taken as important opportunities for continuous improvement learning and another cycle of innovation.

Of course, the dyad in the capacity of health innovators develops strategies and means to avert resistance, promote learning, and engage members in a dialogue about how change creates gains for the organization as a whole. The strong presence of effective middle managers in innovation implementation can support the transformation of hospitals into integrated health systems and the flow of key strategic and clinical information across practice sites and units (Belasen and Rufer 2014).

DIAGNOSING CULTURES

A systematic cultural assessment, such as the one depicted in exhibit 9.2, is a necessary precursor to implementing effective change efforts. Assessments of organizational culture are useful because they help managers and organizations target the trajectory of change and enhance organizational performance. The example in exhibit 9.2 demonstrates the sentiments that members display in expressing a desire to shift from an overemphasis on efficiency to one that incorporates collaboration and innovation.

SURVEY METHODOLOGY

The survey in exhibit 9.3 will allow you to identify your organizational culture, providing a result similar to the chart in exhibit 9.2. Respondents fill out the survey twice—first, as they see the culture of the hospital ("actual"), and second, as they would like to see their culture manifest in the future ("desired"). A simple Excel spreadsheet that lists the responses (or ratings) and a conversion to a radar (or spidergram) chart will help you to create visuals specific to your dyad.

Exhibit 9.2: Cultural Types

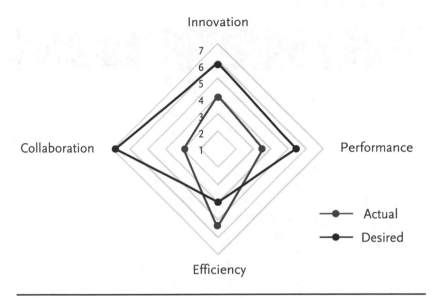

Exhibit 9.3: Survey Methodology for Diagnosing Hospital Culture

Frequency Level (Seven-Point Likert Scale)
Thinking about your healthcare setting, reflect on each statement by indicating the response that best matches your beliefs, first in terms of the actual culture (i.e., current beliefs, expectations, views, behaviors) and desired culture.

1 – *Very untrue of what I believe*
2 – *Untrue of what I believe*
3 – *Somewhat untrue of what I believe*
4 – *Neutral*
5 – *Somewhat true of what I believe*
6 – *True of what I believe*
7 – *Very true of what I believe*

(continued)

Cultural Type	Expectations and Behavioral Indicators	Actual	Desired
Innovation	1. We focus on the human experience to identify design needs.		
	2. We invest time and energy resources in connecting with our patients.		
	3. My hospital incentivizes innovative approaches to healthcare delivery.		
	4. We promote innovation using interfunctional collaboration.		
	5. We value problem solving, brainstorming, and creative thinking.		
	6. We create custom solutions that advance population health.		
	7. My hospital leadership embraces disruptive innovation.		
		AVG	
Performance	8. Quality ratings are an important strategic focus of our health system.		
	9. To grow, we need to compete as an integrated health system.		
	10. The importance of performance measurement and reporting is high.		
	11. Hospital performance measures are viewed through the lens of value.		
	12. Assessing my hospital financial risk position is vital for our success.		
	13. We focus on financial ratio analysis to evaluate hospital performance.		
	14. Operating margins are vital for meeting patient and community needs.		
		AVG	

(continued)

Exhibit 9.3: Survey Methodology for Diagnosing Hospital Culture *(continued)*

Efficiency	15. The hospital leadership uses bureaucratic control to achieve integration.
	16. Our administrative costs are very high.
	17. We rely on bureaucratic lines to maximize efficiencies.
	18. Managerial decision-making in my hospital is top-down.
	19. Hospital leaders draw on positional power to drive goals.
	20. My hospital leadership is more transactional than transformational.
	21. Work units are highly specialized.
	AVG
Collabora-tion	22. We rely on interfunctional collaborative teams.
	23. We focus on interprofessional cooperation to improve patient care.
	24. Healthcare teams interact dynamically to deliver quality services.
	25. Our high-performance teams rely on lateral communication.
	26. We measure our hospitals' commitment to quality care by what leaders do.
	27. Teamwork in our hospital positively affects patient safety.
	28. Teams are effective in reducing errors and improving quality care.
	AVG

The bar chart in exhibit 9.4 is a replica of the spidergram in exhibit 9.2. Both figures demonstrate significant differences between the current profile of the hospital's culture and the preferred culture. Again, the overall trajectory involves a shift from a relative focus on performance and efficiency to a relative focus on collaboration and innovation.

Of course, these cultural types are not exclusive in the sense that they are viewed as binary. Instead, the dyad leaders can look at the trade-offs between the different types, recognize their inherent tensions, and revise or shape the culture based on the desired trajectory.

When the updates to organizational culture are conducted on an ongoing basis, the hospital culture becomes adaptive and, on balance, supportive of the hospital's strategic direction.

Exhibit 9.4: Gaps Between Actual and Desired Cultures

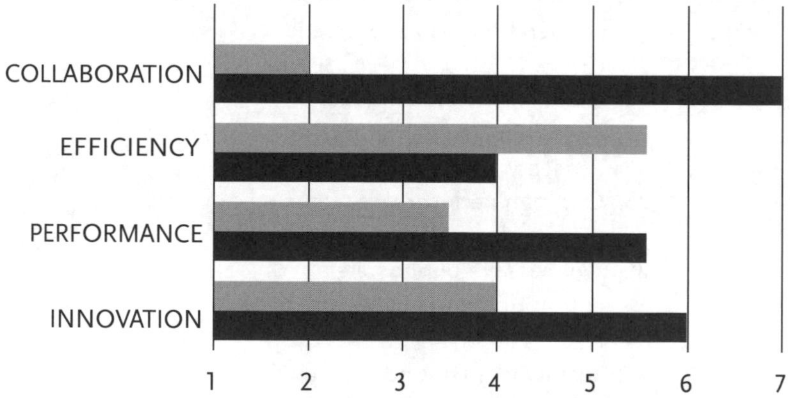

		INNOVATION	PERFORMANCE	EFFICIENCY	COLLABORATION
	Actual	4	3.6	5.5	2
	Desired	6	5.5	4	7

KEY TAKEAWAYS

- The four types of cultures—innovation, performance, efficiency, and collaboration—are consistent with the framework discussed earlier in the book and with the dyad leadership roles.
- Assessments of organizational culture are useful because they help managers and organizations to realign the culture with the new strategic direction.
- When updates to organizational culture are conducted on an ongoing basis, the hospital culture becomes adaptive and, on balance, supportive of the health system's strategic direction.

REFERENCES

Belasen, A. T., and A. R. Belasen. 2016. "Value in the Middle: Cultivating Middle Managers in Healthcare Organizations." *Journal of Management Development* 35 (9): 1149–62.

Belasen, A., and R. Rufer. 2014. "Innovation Communication for Effective Inter-Professional Collaboration: A Stakeholder Perspective." In *Strategy and Communication for Innovation*, 2nd ed., edited by N. Pfeffermann, T. Minshall, and L. Mortara, 227–40. New York: Springer.

Plsek, P. E. 2014. "Creating a Culture of Innovation." Agency for Healthcare Research and Quality. Published April 23. https://innovations.ahrq.gov/article/creating-culture-innovation.

PART III

Role: Value Strategist

Exhibit 3: Value Strategist

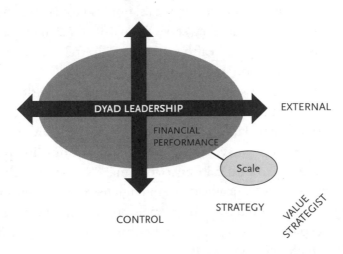

As reimbursements move toward bundled payments and population health, financial incentives and clinical decisions must reflect not only quality but also collaboration, efficiency, use of ancillary personnel, and patient centeredness. Building a platform for hospital–physician collaboration that is robust enough to achieve care that is safe, timely, effective, efficient, and equitable is a prime goal.

To become more accountable, hospital leaders pursue greater operational efficiencies and synergies through economies of scale including mergers and acquisitions. They also advance greater economies of scope through partnerships and coordinated care across groups of providers and specialty clinics inside and outside the integrated system.

A primary objective of the value strategist in a healthcare organization is to invest in an effective electronic health record (EHR) platform that supports the goal of clinical integration, evidence-based care through data collection, analysis, and data sharing to reduce clinical variance, population health, and effective outcomes.

The success of health networks hinges on proactive strategies by dyad leaders to assume greater responsibility, not only for providing medical services or pharmaceuticals, but also for sustaining the health of the populations they serve. Many of the challenges they face in transforming their health systems are interrelated and weigh equally in consideration and impact.

Chapter 10 describes the balanced scorecard and performance indicators for health systems. Chapter 11 provides evidence about the increase in financial burden and slumping Medicare margins, which suppress top-line revenue growth and bottom-line profitability. The drives toward gaining a larger market share or achieving greater efficiency and cost advantage through mergers and consolidation are complemented by strong brand promotion and retention strategies explored in chapter 12 and hospital optimization efforts described in chapter 13.

CHAPTER 10

The Context for the Dyad Value Strategist

INTRODUCTION

Identifying and promoting dyad leaders throughout the health system and ensuring they are on board with the transition toward clinical integration can make or break the postmerger efforts. Because dyad leaders are responsible for the entire continuum of care, they collaborate to identify issues, goals, and outcomes while monitoring variation in both cost and quality. In doing so, they avoid the tendency to only lower the average cost of a procedure or increase the average quality score. This underscores the need to recalibrate scorecard metrics that are based on average performance measures. At the same time, identifying operational measures that ensure financial stability through reimbursement is critical. Hospital leaders must employ tools such as balanced scorecards to create value and to invest in and evaluate internal business processes, patient satisfaction, learning, and innovation.

THE BALANCED SCORECARD

Originated by scholars Robert Kaplan and David Norton (1992), the balanced scorecard (BSC) remains relevant and useful for healthcare leaders working to transcend traditional notions about functional barriers, improve problem solving, and make wise decisions. The BSC links four domains (or quadrants): internal business, innovation and learning, customer perspective, and financial performance. A simplified version of the BSC appears in exhibit 10.1.

The BSC reflects financial, customer satisfaction, internal process, and innovation and improvement activities. Scorecards and dashboards differ in significant ways. Dashboards typically serve as tactical indicators; they use trend lines to focus on processes rather than outcomes. The BSC, on the other hand, is aimed at measuring organizational performance metrics based on benchmarks or strategic goals. These include the following:

- Customer perspective: time, quality, performance, service
- Internal business perspective: cycle time, quality, productivity, costs

Exhibit 10.1: The Balanced Scorecard

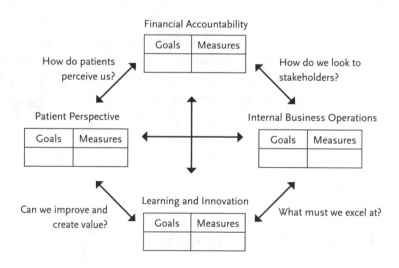

Source: Adapted from Kaplan and Norton (1992).

- Innovation and learning: new products, creation of value for customers, improving operating efficiencies
- Financial perspective: cash flow, sales growth, market share

BSCs facilitate a single dashboard view, in which seemingly unrelated business elements are united under a common focus that provides insight into how well the hospital progresses toward achieving its goals.

GUIDING AWAY FROM SUBOPTIMIZATION

The BSC is consistent with the continuous improvement initiatives underway in many healthcare organizations: clinical integration, patient centeredness, customer–supplier partnership that fosters cost savings and efficiency, and collaboration that benefits all parties. It is also consistent with the Centers for Medicare & Medicaid Services' value-based payment metrics of clinical care, efficiency and cost reduction, and safety. The quadrants in a typical BSC reflect the hospital's key initiatives, including medication safety, operations, quality, finance, research, and education. Examples appear in exhibit 10.2.

Exhibit 10.2: Goals and Measures

Financial Indicators		
Revenue growth	• Growth in net revenues • Volume growth by key service line • Amount and sources of funds raised • Number of contracts received • Percentage of contracts relative to competition • Revenues from new contracts • Patient census	• Market share • Referrals and use • Donors' contributions • Funds raised for facility improvements • Payer mix • Number of outpatient visits • Research grants • Financial growth rate • Strategic expansion budgeting

(continued)

Productivity	• Profit • Operating margin • Depreciation • Amortization and expense as a percentage of net revenue • Total assets by net revenue • Cost per case • Cost per discharge	• Supply expense and pharmacy expense • Personnel cost • Reduced cash • Efficiency ratios such as overtime use • Unit expenditures • Length of stay • Operating room supply expense per surgical case

Patient Indicators

Patient satisfaction	• Patient complaints • Patient referral rate • Percentage of patients recommending the hospital • Waiting time • Access • Accurate diagnosis rate	• Incidents (including falls, medication errors) • Hospital-acquired conditions • Discharge timeliness • Preventable readmissions • Hospital cleanliness
Customer acquisition	• New contracts per period • Increase in market share	
Stakeholder satisfaction	• Number of health maintenance organization contracts • Number of complaints • Information sharing among stakeholders (e.g., number of responses)	• Number of referrals • Increased donations
Employee satisfaction	• Employee satisfaction • Physician satisfaction • Nurses' retention rate	• Employee turnover rate • Absenteeism rate

Internal Business Operations Indicators

Operational Indicators	• Length of stay • Case cancellations • Waiting time • Discharge • Readmission rate • Mortality rate • Number of patient falls	• Claim processing accuracy • Patient complaints • Percentage of emergency department patients triaged within 15 minutes of arrival • Billing and collection ratios

(continued)

Safety	• Infection rate • Coding error rate (clinic and hospital)	• Medication errors per dose • Occupational injuries • Restraint usage
Productivity	• Cost per capita • Cost per diagnosis • Cost per product • Staffing	• Utilization • Percentage of occupied beds • Hours per unit of activity • Resource usage
Innovation	• Product innovation • Staff training • Number of physicians using electronic health record (EHR)	• Development of employee knowledge
Learning and Innovation Indicators		
Human capital	• Staff development • Dollars spent on training and development • Continuing education credits per full-time employee	• Publications • Tuition reimbursement per year
Technology	• EHR implementation • Informatics training	• Work design • Interoperability training
Continuous improvement	• New service lines • New research projects	• Number of partners participating in joint projects
Organization capital	• Leadership development • Cultural survey results • Communication assessment	• Employee motivation and empowerment • Number of interprofessional collaborations

When designed properly and updated in a timely manner, the BSC can present a broad view of the hospital's performance, serve as a guide for strategic decision-making, and improve the quality of medical services. By linking measures of financial outcomes, patient care, and reliability of internal processes with innovation and organizational learning, the tool helps hospital leaders to guard against suboptimization. Dyad leaders review possible trade-offs across a number of goals and measures and take proactive steps to balance four elements: regulation with innovation, and patient experience and quality care with financial investment and performance management.

It is important to note that different health systems use different variants of the BSC to map their unique mission, goals, strategies, and measures. For example, Sunnybrook Health Sciences Centre's (2019) strategic mapping includes three main dimensions: quality of patient care, research and education, and accountability and sustainability.

Another example is Humber River Hospital's (2019) BSC, which includes four dimensions (and several measures):

1. Stakeholders (overall rating of care, community consultation)
2. Learning and growth (retention, leadership development)
3. Financial and accountability (percentage of beds occupied by patients who could have been receiving care elsewhere, ED wait time)
4. Internal processes (infection prevention, mortality rates, surgical safety checklist compliance)

STRATEGIC VALUE

Dyad leaders, who balance their clinical responsibilities with administrative roles while serving as value strategists, can help inspire the transformation toward a value-based health system and mobilize support for that vision.

Unlike tactical dashboards, which focus on processes, the BSC is strategic, with performance metrics based on benchmarks or strategic goals. The BSC presents a broader view of the hospital's performance and serves as a guide for improving the quality of medical services. Increasing efficiency and promoting value is achieved by the following actions:

- Enhancing the alignment between physicians and administrators to create new value
- Improving operating costs and functionality by streamlining operations, reducing waste, and eliminating unnecessary errors and redundancies
- Transitioning away from the traditional fee-for-service payment model
- Transcending organizational boundaries and silos by adopting strategic views and tools such as the BSC
- Increasing the institution's focus on risk management and patient safety
- Promoting clinical, financial, operational, technological, and cultural alignment
- Expanding revenue cycle management by improving operating efficiencies and focusing more on quality of care and improvement of medical outcomes
- Rationalizing the system through external affiliations, partnerships, and consolidation of service lines to achieve greater synergies and provide cost-effective services
- Allocating capital to improve EHR implementation for the dissemination and sharing of data
- Employing analytics to measure financial and quality performance on a continuous basis
- Engaging local leaders across the clinical integration network with a strong focus on cost efficiency and coordinated care
- Hiring care professionals and technology specialists to build high-quality teams
- Ensuring development of effective postdischarge plans to improve outcomes and reduce costly readmissions

KEY TAKEAWAYS

- The BSC provides some level of transparency to hospitals and communities.
- It provides a powerful framework for identifying and communicating a successful strategy.
- This tool aligns the health system goals and means to achieve them.
- It allows dyad leaders to measure the value of the business strategy of the four perspectives from the larger context that also includes clinical and nonclinical assessments.
- The BSC links tangible outcomes with financial obligations.
- It reminds executives that in addition to tracking financial metrics, tracking quality and service is also important.
- It promotes a dialogue to increase quality and promote joint accountability.

REFERENCES

Humber River Hospital. 2019. "Balanced Scorecard." Accessed March 1. www.coursehero.com/tutors-problems/Business/9148427 -Review-the-balanced-scorecard-for-Humber-River-Hospital-Give -some-exa/.

Kaplan, R. S., and D. P. Norton. 1992. "The Balanced Scorecard: Measures That Drive Performance." *Harvard Business Review* 70 (1): 71–79.

Sunnybrook Health Sciences Centre. 2019. "Balanced Scorecard and Patient Safety Indicators." Accessed March 1. https:// sunnybrook.ca/scorecard/.

CHAPTER 11

Operating Margins

INTRODUCTION

Hospitals face considerable increases in uncompensated care, which represses top-line revenue growth and bottom-line profitability. The payment a hospital receives for the service it provides depends on the type of payer. Governmental payers, including Medicare and Medicaid, set rates, and most hospitals, lacking bargaining power compared to commercial plans, accept government rates to have access to these patients.

In general, hospitals lose money on Medicare and Medicaid patients, but offset their losses by charging private insurers more. However, a growing proportion of Medicare business puts considerable strain on hospital revenues. Medicare expenditures will continue to grow at double-digit rates through 2021 as the baby boomer population ages. This chapter covers the challenges associated with low margins resulting from payment rate differentials, which reflects the disproportionate amount of revenue coming from government.

LOW MARGINS

According to Moody's, Medicare payments increased from 44.9 percent of median gross revenue to 45.6 percent in fiscal year (FY) 2017, and Medicaid increased from 15 percent to 15.5 percent. The median commercial insurance rate declined to 31.9 percent from 32.6 percent (Moody's Investor Services 2018). The proportion of commercial payers, which, in effect, subsidizes the cost of Medicare and Medicaid, will continue to shift downward in the future. This trend will most likely continue, especially if the benefits from the Medicaid expansion authorized in the Affordable Care Act (ACA) will not be fully materialized by states that did not implement the expansion, leaving many without an affordable coverage option.

A central goal of the ACA is to reduce significantly the number of uninsured individuals by providing a continuum of affordable coverage options through Medicaid and health insurance marketplaces. The ACA expands Medicaid coverage to adults with income up to 138 percent of the federal poverty level (FPL). Following the June 2012 Supreme Court ruling, states faced a decision about whether to adopt the Medicaid expansion. It is important to note that, per Centers for Medicare & Medicaid Services guidelines, there is no deadline for states to implement the Medicaid expansion (Kaiser Family Foundation 2019). As of early 2019, 14 states had not adopted the expansion.

The ACA mandated that Medicaid disproportionate-share hospital (DSH) funds be cut by $43 billion between FYs 2018 and 2025. However, Congress delayed the cuts, which were supposed to start in 2014, after hospitals warned that increased patient volume fell below uncompensated-care costs. Between 2013 and 2014, total hospital uncompensated care for Medicaid-enrolled and uninsured patients fell by about $4.6 billion, or 9.3 percent, with the largest declines in states that expanded Medicaid, where uncompensated care costs were $10.8 billion in 2014—down $5.7 billion, or 35 percent, from 2013 (the year before ACA coverage expansions took full effect). Medicaid DSH payments totaled $18 billion in FY 2014 (Medicaid and CHIP Payment and Access Commission 2017). By 2015, uncompensated care portions fell significantly in expansion states, from 3.9 percent in 2013–2014 to 2.3 percent of operating costs (Dranove, Garthwaite, and Ody 2017).

GREATER FINANCIAL BURDEN

The American Health Care Act (AHCA), passed by the US House of Representatives in May 2017, is likely to increase uncompensated care costs in the future and trigger lower operating margins at health systems, including those in the 31 states that expanded Medicaid under the ACA (Haught et al. 2017). These hospitals could see a 78 percent increase in uncompensated care costs between 2017 and 2026, even though the law restores Medicaid DSH hospital payments.

Hospitals in Medicaid expansion states may experience a 14 percent drop in Medicaid revenues between 2017 and 2026, compared to a 3 percent anticipated reduction among hospitals in the 19 states that did not expand. Rural hospitals in Medicaid expansion states, on average, could experience an 18 percent decline in Medicaid payments, and rural hospitals in nonexpansion states could face negative margins of 3.3 percent.

Hospitals in 28 of the states that have expanded Medicaid are expected to have negative operating margins under the AHCA by 2026. A few examples include Louisiana (–4.2 percent), West Virginia (–6.8 percent), Arizona (–6.0 percent), and Ohio (–1.8 percent). Hospitals in nonexpansion states such as Maine (–10.3 percent) and Nebraska (–5.5 percent) also are projected to have negative operating margins in 2026. Operating margins for hospitals across the states are likely to drop to –5.3 percent in 2026 under the AHCA.

THE CONGRESSIONAL BUDGET OFFICE'S NEW ESTIMATES

In the fall of 2017, the Congressional Budget Office (CBO) released a report about the budgetary effects of options for a premium support system (CBO 2017). The intent was to highlight the potential reduction in federal spending with the assumption that the system would be implemented in 2022. Future cost estimates for legislative proposals could differ substantially from the 2017 estimates.

In the options the CBO analyzed, the federal government's contribution would be determined from insurers' bids, in which Medicare's traditional fee-for-service (FFS) program would be included as a competing plan. CBO examined two options for determining the federal contribution: one would set the contribution based on the second-lowest bid in each region; the other would use the region's average bid. The CBO also examined the effects of grandfathering, which would keep beneficiaries in the current Medicare program if they were eligible for Medicare before the premium support system took effect, instead of requiring all beneficiaries to enter the premium support system once it began. In a premium support system, the federal government would provide a set, monthly payment on behalf of each eligible Medicare beneficiary to be applied toward the purchase of health insurance—either a private plan, a Medicare Advantage plan, or traditional Medicare.

The CBO's new estimates indicate the following:

- Without grandfathering, the second-lowest-bid option would reduce net federal spending for Medicare by $419 billion between 2022 and 2026; the average-bid option would reduce such spending by $184 billion. See estimated differences in exhibit 11.1.
- With grandfathering, the second-lowest-bid option would reduce net federal spending for Medicare by $50 billion between 2022 and 2026; the average-bid option would reduce such spending by $21 billion.

Those savings would arise because private insurers' bids would generally be lower than FFS costs per capita and would substantially influence the federal contribution. Savings would be much smaller if the options included a grandfathering provision because only a small portion of the Medicare population would be covered by the new system initially; that portion would increase gradually.

Exhibit 11.1: Estimated Differences from Outcomes Under Current Law, Without Grandfathering, in 2024

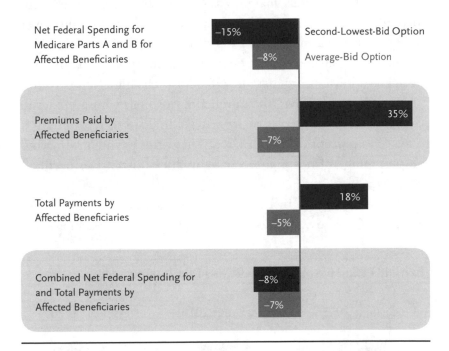

Source: Reprinted from CBO (2017).

These cuts would increase the financial risk on health providers and insurers, raise per capita caps, and reduce the ability of health-care providers to care for older, sicker, and disabled populations. They may also strain the ability of states to control costs and sustain managed care payments (Morse 2017).

SLUMPING MEDICARE MARGINS

In 2011, the average hospital margin on Medicare patients (a mea-sure of the relationship between Medicare payments for Medicare patients and the cost of their care at hospitals) was –5 percent. The total margins for hospitals, however, dipped to –6.5 percent in 2012. In 2013, hospital all-payer margins were a record low: –7.2 percent.

In 2013, the hospitals' margin was –5.4 percent. Relatively efficient hospitals (i.e., hospitals with lower costs and better quality over three years) had a margin of 2 percent in 2013. In 2014, hospitals posted a –5.8 percent margin on their Medicare business. In 2015, the aggregate Medicare margin across hospitals hit a –7.1 percent.

As exhibit 11.2 shows, the number of hospitals whose Medicare payments were reduced grew from 1,235 in 2016 to 1,343 in 2017. In 2016, 59 percent of hospitals received bonus payments; in 2017, the percentage of hospital receiving financial incentives declined to 54 percent.

On the aggregate, in 2016, both Medicare and Medicaid payments fell below costs, with combined underpayments reaching $68.8

Exhibit 11.2: Hospital Value-Based Purchasing

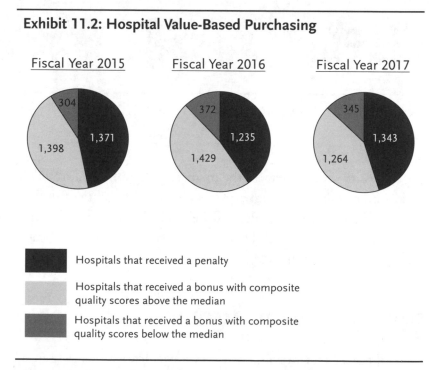

Fiscal Year 2015   Fiscal Year 2016   Fiscal Year 2017

■ Hospitals that received a penalty

▨ Hospitals that received a bonus with composite quality scores above the median

▨ Hospitals that received a bonus with composite quality scores below the median

Source: Data from US Government Accountability Office (2017).

billion, a shortfall of $48.8 billion for Medicare and $20.0 billion for Medicaid. During that year, for Medicare, hospitals received payments of only 87 cents for every dollar spent caring for Medicare patients in 2016.

For Medicaid, hospitals received payment of only 88 cents for every dollar spent by hospitals caring for Medicaid patients. Furthermore, in 2016, 66 percent of hospitals received Medicare payments less than cost, while 61 percent of hospitals received Medicaid payments less than cost (American Hospital Association 2017). Margins were expected to drop to –10 percent in 2017 (MedPAC 2017).

Margins Hit 10-Year Record Low

A new Moody's report shows nonprofit and public hospitals' margins have hit a 10-year low, falling below levels seen during the last recession.

"Despite positive volume trends, we expect expense pressures, declining reimbursement and a shifting payer mix will contribute to challenged financial performance over the next year," the report said.

Profitability margins hit the lowest point in a decade, with median operating cash flow margins dipping to 8.1 percent from 9.5 percent in 2016, and lower-rated hospitals felt a significant strain on margins. These facilities are usually smaller with fragile financial operations making them more vulnerable to industry pressures. They also have less negotiating power with insurers and a tougher time attracting physicians. This vulnerability will likely fuel additional merger and acquisition activity as these facilities struggle to survive.

—Beth Jones Sanborn (2018)

POWER DYNAMICS AND SHIFTING COSTS

With commercial payers, hospitals are able to negotiate rates based on expected volume, although size and market power of both parties matter. For example, in 2016, leveraging their bargaining power through consolidation allowed Dignity Health and Sutter Health, the two largest hospital networks in northern California, to shift costs by setting prices 25 percent higher than other hospitals in the state. However, in March 2018, California's attorney general announced a lawsuit against Sutter Health, alleging the hospital giant engaged in anticompetitive conduct that drove up prices for patients and employers (Terhune 2018).

Offsetting a cut in Medicare and Medicaid reimbursement with a rate increase from private insurers may work for the larger health systems, as market power undercuts insurers' ability to negotiate prices. With the backup of economies of scale, hospital systems with significant market power are often able to negotiate higher payment rates from commercial insurers—as high as 50 percent above their costs and even 75 percent or higher than Medicare rates (MedPAC 2016).

The bigger the health insurer, the lower the prices it can negotiate from physician groups. Moreover, commercial rates are often determined based on a percentage of Medicare or some other formula that private insurers use based on Medicare rates. Therefore, cuts to Medicare rates may have a larger impact on hospital finances than just among Medicare patients.

Smaller community health centers lack volume or bargaining power to secure advantageous arrangements with plans. Private insurers set predetermined rates on a "take it or leave it" basis. Institutions in urban areas are particularly vulnerable, as plans with sufficient numbers of primary care providers can exclude them or can simply determine unfavorable rates.

CONTROLLING COSTS AND BLURRING LINES

As healthcare systems and physician groups have been willing to assume greater financial risks for their patients, provider-owned health plans (POHPs) have also become larger to manage value-based care agreements and capitated payment contracts more effectively. POHPs allow the network to leverage local or geographic economies of scale and skill. For example, in 2015, San Francisco–based Dignity Health Provider Resources sought a license to enter into contracts with financial risk for the full spectrum of a patient's care (Evans 2015).

Between 2010 and 2014, the number of providers in the United States offering at least one health plan grew to 106, amounting to a 3 percent annual increase. Total enrollment grew 6 percent annually over that same period, from 12.4 million in 2010 to 15.3 million in 2014 (Abrams and Phillips 2016). The total number of POHPs increased from 256 in 2015 to 268 in 2016. Membership in these plans increased from 32.8 million to 36.3 million. By 2017, about 300 plans owned by health systems operated in the marketplace (Morse 2016).

As insurers, these POHPs face incentives to control costs. Integration makes it easier to share information about patients and track quality, which improves the ability of the health network to manage patients with chronic conditions. Perhaps the biggest risk POHPs face involves the inherent tension between payer value creation and provider value creation: Payers create value by negotiating reduced reimbursement rates with providers, lowering utilization rates, or both. By contrast, providers create value through pricing and by increasing asset usage. As discussed earlier in the book, some providers have also focused on higher-margin procedures. Health systems that want to benefit from having a health plan must be proactive in reconciling these differences in value creation (Khanna, Smith, and Sutaria 2015).

Risks to Providers of Starting a Plan

Once they join a provider-owned insurer, high-cost patients shift from being revenue generators to liabilities. A successful plan needs to attract enrollees from outside the system. . . . Due to their small scale and unique structure, provider-owned insurers may have to pay more for reinsurance to protect against large losses. These costs may erode the savings from eliminating insurers [or intermediaries] as middlemen between providers and patients. Health systems that become insurers also risk creating a more antagonistic relationship with traditional insurers, who are now competitors. For example, Blue Cross Blue Shield of Nebraska excluded Catholic Health's hospitals from its provider network for 10 months after Catholic proposed to start selling insurance in the state. Catholic Health exited the insurance market in early 2017.

Employers prefer to contract with insurers that have provider networks that are accessible to all of their employees. . . . Provider-owned insurers with only a handful of clinic locations will have trouble competing in the group insurance market. Provider-owned insurers can expand their geographic reach by contracting with unaffiliated providers, but then they forgo the benefits of integration. Smaller provider-owned insurers will be at a disadvantage relative to large commercial insurers when negotiating reimbursement rates with outside physicians and hospitals. . . . The ability of provider-owned insurers to attract enrollees and obtain favorable treatment from regulators hinges on their ability to cut costs.

—David H. Howard and Erin E. Trish (2017)

Mergers are an attractive way to achieve greater reach outside a health system's standard market segment; they are also great for expanding network capacity. However, they face legal challenges in building competitive provider networks. Advocate Health Care and NorthShore University HealthSystem walked away from plans to merge after a US district judge granted a request by the Federal Trade Commission and the state of Illinois for a preliminary injunction to stop them temporarily (Schencker 2017).

When forming a POHP, dyad leaders should consider four areas of questions (Khanna, Smith, and Sutaria 2015):

1. Strategy
   - What strategy are we focusing on and where will the incremental value created by the POHP come from?
   - Which of the market segments offer the best option for expanding the network?
   - What type of health plan will we offer?
   - How can we best leverage the integrated network?
   - How do the potential benefits compare with those obtained through a closer partnership with local payers?
   - What are the risks?
2. Structure and Function
   - How should the POHP be structured to manage the tension between payer and provider?
   - How should we handle the conflict between the POHP and third-party plans?
   - What is the optimal way to organize the combined entity (e.g., geography, customer segment)?
   - Who should lead the different parts?
   - Which part of the organization should own specific business processes?

3. Operational, Financial, and Regulatory Issues
    • How should the POHP get ready, and what investment is required?
    • In what key areas do we need additional skills or capabilities (e.g., member acquisition, regulatory and compliance, utilization management)?
    • How do we manage the balance sheet risk of the combined payer–provider entity?
    • How much capital is required to build an appropriate infrastructure and sustain the appropriate risk-based capital levels?

KEY TAKEAWAYS

• A growing proportion of Medicare and Medicaid expenditures have put considerable strain on hospital revenues. In 2016, underpayments by Medicare and Medicaid combined reached $68.8 billion.
• The number of hospitals whose Medicare payments were reduced grew from 1,235 in 2016 to 1,343 in 2017. In 2016, 59 percent of hospitals received bonus payments; in 2017, the percentage of hospitals receiving financial incentives fell to 54 percent.
• With the backup of economies of scale, larger hospital systems are able to negotiate higher payment rates from commercial insurers, as high as 50 percent above their costs and even 75 percent or higher than Medicare rates.
• As insurers, POHPs face incentives to control costs. Integration makes it easier to share information about patients, track quality, and manage patients with chronic conditions.
• Employers prefer to contract with insurers that have provider networks that are accessible to all of their employees across geographical areas.

REFERENCES

Abrams, M. N., and G. Phillips. 2016. "Taking the Leap into Coverage." *Trustee Magazine.* Published September 12. www .trusteemag.com/articles/1129-provider-owned-health-plans.

American Hospital Association. 2017. "Underpayment by Medicare and Medicaid Fact Sheet." Published December. www.aha .org/system/files/2018-01/medicaremedicaidunderpmt%20 2017.pdf.

Congressional Budget Office (CBO). 2017. *A Premium Support System for Medicare: Updated Analysis of Illustrative Options.* Published October. www.cbo.gov/publication/53077.

Dranove, D., C. Garthwaite, and C. Ody. 2017. "The Impact of the ACA's Medicaid Expansion on Hospitals' Uncompensated Care Burden and the Potential Effects of Repeal." Commonwealth Fund. Published May 3. www.commonwealthfund.org/ publications/issue-briefs/2017/may/impact-acas-medicaid -expansion-hospitals-uncompensated-care.

Evans, M. 2015. "Dignity Health Will Seek License to Assume Financial Risk for Patients." *Modern Healthcare.* Published February 27. www.modernhealthcare.com/article/20150227/ NEWS/150229912/dignity-health-will-seek-license-to-assume -financial-risk-for-patients.

Haught, R., A. Dobson, J. DaVanzo, and M. K. Abrams. 2017. "How the American Health Care Act's Changes to Medicaid Will Affect Hospital Finances in Every State." The Commonwealth Fund. Published June 23. www.commonwealthfund.org/publications/ blog/2017/jun/how-changes-to-medicaid-will-affect-hospital -finances-in-every-state.

Howard, D. H., and E. Trish. 2017. "Provider-Owned Insurers." *American Journal of Managed Care.* Published September 13. www.ajmc.com/journals/issue/2017/2017-vol23-n9/provider -owned-insurers.

Kaiser Family Foundation. 2019. "Status of State Action on the Medicaid Expansion Decision." Updated February 13. www.kff.org/health-reform/state-indicator/state-activity-around-expanding-medicaid-under-the-affordable-care-act.

Khanna, G., E. Smith, and S. Sutaria. 2015. "Provider-Led Health Plans: The Next Frontier—or the 1990s All Over Again?" McKinsey & Company. Published November 12. https://healthcare.mckinsey.com/sites/default/files/Provider-led%20health%20plans.pdf.

Medicaid and CHIP Payment and Access Commission. 2017. "Analyzing Disproportionate Share Hospital Allotments to States." In *MACStats: Medicaid and CHIP Data Book*. Published March. www.macpac.gov/wp-content/uploads/2017/03/Analyzing-Disproportionate-Share-Hospital-Allotments-to-States.pdf.

Medicare Payment Advisory Commission (MedPAC). 2017. "Medicare and the Health Care Delivery System." Published June 18. www.medpac.gov/-documents-/reports.

———. 2016. "Meeting Highlight: Hospital Consolidation and Its Implications for Medicare." Published November 15. http://medpac.gov/-blog-/medpacblog/2016/11/15/meeting-highlight-hospital-consolidation-and-its-implications-for-medicare.

Moody's Investor Services. 2018. "Research Announcement: Moody's—US NFP and Public Hospitals' Annual Medians Show Expense Growth Topping Revenues for Second Year." Published August 28. www.moodys.com/research/Moodys-US-NFP-public-hospitals-annual-medians-show-expense-growth--PBM_1139331.

Morse, S. 2017. "Billions in Proposed Budget Cuts to Medicare, Medicaid Threaten Provider Compensation." *Healthcare Finance*. Published October 23. www.healthcarefinancenews.com/news/billions-proposed-budget-cuts-medicare-medicaid-threaten-provider-compensation.

———. 2016. "25 Biggest Provider-Sponsored Health Plans Include Some of the Nation's Biggest Systems." Published September 13. www.healthcarefinancenews.com/news/25 -biggest-provider-sponsored-health-plans-include-some-nations -biggest-systems.

Sanborn, B. J. 2018. "Nonprofit, Public Hospital Margins Hit 10-Year Record Low, Moody's Report Says." *Healthcare Finance.* Published April 24. www.healthcarefinancenews.com/news/ nonprofit-public-hospital-margins-hit-10-year-record-low -moodys-report-says.

Schencker, L. 2017. "NorthShore, Advocate Drop Merger Plan After Judge's Ruling." *Chicago Tribune.* Published March 7. www.chicagotribune.com/business/ct-advocate-northshore -merger-decision-0308-biz-20170307-story.html.

Terhune, C. 2018. "California Sues Hospital Giant Sutter Health, Where Study Found Prices 25% Higher." *USA Today.* Published March 30. www.usatoday.com/story/news/ nation/2018/03/30/sutter-health-lawsuit-california-hospital -consolidation/474742002/.

US Government Accountability Office. 2017. "Hospital Value-Based Purchasing: CMS Should Take Steps to Ensure Lower Quality Hospitals Do Not Qualify for Bonuses." Published June 30. www.gao.gov/products/GAO-17-551.

CHAPTER 12

Brand Promotion and Retention

INTRODUCTION

Providing high-quality, effective, and efficient healthcare while building competitive and sustainable integrated health services requires branding and promotion strategies linked with population health capabilities and localized clinics, patient engagement, and targeted outreach.

To deliver safe, high-quality care while simultaneously achieving a sustainable competitive advantage requires partnership and collaboration with physicians, community health centers, long-term and post-acute care facilities, inpatient rehabilitation facilities, home and community-based services, skilled nursing facilities, and a host of other social services. As the pressure toward a value-based, integrated care continuum is mounting, cooperative marketing opportunities will begin to present themselves. This includes strategic positioning and market analysis involving many stakeholders, including allied health services, competing hospitals, physician practices, and health plans.

Dyad leaders must recognize the need to engage partners in strategic marketing initiatives, especially in light of the trend to facilitate the movement of patients across the continuum of care. Successful health systems develop cooperative marketing and branding strategies, which not only extend their limited marketing resources but also reach out to populations and accomplish their strategic objectives effectively.

BUILDING CRITICAL MASS

Physician-owned specialty hospitals are not distributed evenly across geographical regions. Many do not have emergency departments (EDs), nurses on duty, or physicians on call. Top-paying medical specialties include orthopedic surgery, cardiology (invasive), cardiology (noninvasive), gastroenterology, urology, hematology and oncology, dermatology, radiology, pulmonology, and general surgery. Even in diagnosis-related groups, profits for doctors can vary because of differences in the severity of patients' conditions (Kaplan 2019). Specializing in highly selective and profitable service lines allows specialty hospitals to build a critical mass of patients and sustain economies of skill and scale.

Full-service hospitals, on the other hand, are vital to meeting the healthcare needs of the communities they serve. They provide a wide range of acute care and diagnostic services, as well as short-term medical treatment for patients, including psychiatric care, substance abuse treatment, AIDS services, emergency services, trauma center treatment, obstetric care, and so on. Unlike single-specialty medical groups, full-service hospitals are struggling in a vicious cycle of declining resources and patient volumes. They suffer from a diminished ability to offer high-quality care and to serve those members of their communities most in need (Baghai, Levin, and Sutaria 2008).

Median operating cash-flow margins, a key measure of profitability, dropped from 9.5 percent in 2016 to 8.1 percent in 2017 as a result of high labor costs and lower reimbursement from commercial and federal payers (Lovelace 2018). To fight back, hospitals have begun to invest in services that deliver profits. Departments such as neurosurgery or interventional cardiology account for a large share of hospital revenues and earnings, in essence subsidizing the unprofitable (yet needed) services. Other health systems invested in hybrid operating rooms (ORs), which integrate image-guided interventional technology. According to Transparency Market Research (2019), the hybrid OR global market value is projected to increase from $661.8 billion in 2017 to $828 billion by 2022. Moreover, the demand for intraoperative diagnostic imaging systems is expected to rise at a significant rate during the forecast period, with sizeable demand in North America.

STRATEGIC CONSIDERATIONS

Good strategy links the organization's mission to its actions, but good strategy also links actions to important organizational goals. For example, in an effort to provide coordinated care to its patients, a community hospital may acquire a medical practice in its primary service area to expand its strategic scope and skills (Belasen, Eisenberg, and Huppertz 2015). Such a move also accomplishes the goal of enhancing the system's market share by virtually ensuring that a very high proportion of inpatient admissions (and revenue from ancillary services like labs, imaging, and medications) will originate from this medical group. Thus, the hospital captures more of the market's healthcare business in two ways:

1. Providing primary care through a medical practice (upstream)
2. Obtaining a higher proportion of the specialty referrals and inpatient admissions (downstream)

No two organizations are exactly alike, and each faces a different situation, both internally and externally. Not every healthcare organization has a dominant market share, nor do all institutions face a fragmented, competitive market. A thorough analysis of the market position is required to properly set goals.

Consider the following scenarios. In scenario A, a hospital health system is located in a rural area, 50 miles away from a medium-sized metropolitan area of two million people. In its service area, it has a large market share but low population density. The population is not growing, and the average age is increasing. While the town is within the media reach of the metro area and people see ads for hospitals there, the area is less attractive to outside competitors.

In scenario B, a hospital health system is located in the middle of a major metropolitan area of six million people with high population density. Many competitors surround it, so it operates in a highly differentiated and competitive market. This hospital has a low market share. The population is highly diverse, the market is growing, and the healthcare needs of the area are growing, too. Clearly, these two organizations face dramatically different situations, much of which their executives do not control. Neither health system can influence the number of people who live in its service area, nor can it affect the age or demographic attributes of its population.

The systems cannot dictate the general economic conditions of their market because of a number of interrelated factors. These include urban mobility (people move out when jobs are scarce, and they move in when the local economy is growing), payer mix (stronger economic conditions mean higher employment, translating to larger numbers of insured patients), and community health (areas with higher unemployment rates usually see different health problems than regions with full employment—e.g., socioeconomic stress and drug consumption).

They also cannot control their services areas' population density— one is in a rural area, and one is urban. The denser the population in a region is, the more intense the competing services will be. While they may have similar missions, these two health systems' strategic goals differ from one another to reflect the reality of the market dynamics each faces.

In scenario A, the health system has the opportunity to become the dominant healthcare provider for the service area, so its goals may include expanding its scope of operations and vertically integrating to provide all the healthcare services needed by the people who live there. Thus, its executives may choose to acquire the region's primary care and specialty medical practices, as well as ancillary services that support the system. Downstream goals will be required to integrate these services into a coherent and effective system, and strategies must be carefully developed to accomplish this goal, down to the unit level.

The health system in scenario B faces an entirely different set of challenges. Because of the size and nature of its market, it could decide to *narrow* its scope of operations to achieve competitive advantage, as it may see opportunities to establish leadership in a niche. For example, based on its relative strengths and the capabilities of its competitors, the health system's leaders could choose to develop specialty service lines such as orthopedics or women's health, allocating resources to build up these areas and differentiate them from the competition.

Downstream strategies would be devised around the goal of defining the health system as a leader in a narrow field. These strategies would include, for instance, building referral relationships and networks so that the primary care providers and specialists would think of this health system's services first and regard them as the best. It would not be necessary to acquire primary care practices to ensure this referral flow, because in a densely populated metropolitan area, there would be too many primary care practices; the health system's service lines would represent a small proportion of a primary care practice's referrals.

Note that such a strategy would not work for the system in scenario A because its market is too small to support a niche strategy. By pursuing a goal to narrow its focus, the health system in scenario B has the opportunity to build a critical mass by capitalizing on its core competencies.

Both scenarios require a great deal of thinking and planning by the boards of directors and executives who lead those systems. The planning effort relies on data and information about the external market and internal capabilities, but perhaps more important, it relies on the insights that the leaders can derive from their careful and thoughtful study of the business.

EXCESS CAPACITY

Studies show that perceived healthcare service quality has an impact on overall patient satisfaction (Belasen and Belasen 2018). Hospitals that can offer high-quality treatments or services attract a greater volume of professional referrals, reduce customer acquisition costs, and sustain their revenue cycle. A reliable and continuing stream of inbound patient referrals from other medical, dental, or professional sources is the lifeblood of many specialty medical groups.

To increase their attractiveness further, hospitals and their affiliated physicians invest in cutting-edge technologies and specialized medical equipment, which they then try to use to recover costs. Buying expensive equipment, however, accelerates excess hospital capacity and continues to motivate hospital executives to reduce unnecessary cost and utilization.

Rising prices, not utilization, drive up healthcare spending across various categories of services. Unnecessary, expensive care amounts to hundreds of billions of dollars in waste, so payers and policymakers have tried to set guidelines for appropriate use (Allen 2017). The Food and Drug Administration, for example, has adopted appropriate-use criteria in an effort to promote institutions' efforts to improve imaging appropriateness.

The National Committee for Quality Assurance's (NCQA) Healthcare Effectiveness Data and Information Set has also determined that overuse of magnetic resonance imaging (MRI) by providers is a *negative* indicator of quality. The NCQA benchmark for the appropriate treatment of low-back pain, for example, is "the percentage of members with a primary diagnosis of low-back pain who did not have an imaging study" (plain X-ray, MRI, CT scan) within 28 days of the diagnosis" (National Committee for Quality Assurance 2012).

HOSPITAL–PHYSICIAN ALIGNMENT

Hospital–physician alignment is one in which a physician obtains privileges to provide medical services in return for income and security, as well as the capacity to provide high-quality care to her patients. The hospital must ensure that

Radiation Safety Appropriate Use

The 2014 RAND Corporation report on the Medicare Imaging Demonstration (MID) project suggested that between 4% and 26% of imaging studies that could be evaluated were inappropriate. . . .The RAND report also reviewed a number of published reports of decision support system (DSS) use. A DSS synthesizes existing evidence on the effectiveness of each procedure, including appropriateness criteria developed by physician specialty societies. . . . A DSS provides immediate feedback to the physician on the appropriateness of a test or treatment ordered for a patient. After the introduction of a DSS to aid physicians in selecting an appropriate examination, the rate of inappropriate examinations decreased in most published reports. DSS can improve the likelihood of appropriateness even when the vast majority of studies are already appropriate. For example, at Massachusetts General Hospital, the percentage of "low utility" studies decreased from 6% to 2% after the introduction of a DSS.

—US Food and Drug Administration (2017)

- appointment wait times are reasonable,
- paperwork is minimal,
- service is of the utmost quality, and
- communication with staff and the referring physician are good.

Creating value for the participants in this exchange relationship is a win–win. When these provisions are not present, however, relationships may become contentious. Physicians can bypass the hospital by sending their patients to competing hospitals. They can open their own diagnostic centers or add ambulatory surgery centers and other services that offer lower costs and easier access than the hospital provides. When doctors take these actions, hospitals may engage in counterstrategies designed to protect their interests. These strategies trigger tacit or even actual conflicts with the hospitals' own physicians. Amid this relationship of simultaneous competition and interdependency, the relationships between hospitals and physicians are fraught with economic and legal risks, contributing to already-high levels of stress and feelings of burnout.

Another challenge involves internal competition over limited resources. For example, if a hospital recruits new orthopedic surgeons for its ORs, these new doctors directly affect the existing orthopedic surgeons' operating room schedules. They will also affect the diagnostic services and physical therapy provided in the hospital. The dual challenge of promoting engagement while overcoming stress is paramount for sustaining hospital–physician alignment.

More Than Half of US Physicians Burned Out, New Study Finds

Nearly two-thirds of U.S. physicians report feeling burned out (42%), depressed (15%) or both (14%), according to a new Medscape survey of 15,000 practicing physicians.

In addition, 33% of respondents stated these depressive feelings affect their relations with patients.

To alleviate burnout, 56% of respondents suggested fewer bureaucratic tasks and 39% suggested fewer hours spent working. About one-third of physicians suggested more money and a more manageable work schedule.

—Jeff Byers (2018)

Ultimately, successful hospital–physician alignment must be more than economic in nature. It must have measurable expectations, mutually shared by the hospital and physicians. The overarching goal must remain the same—to improve the quality and efficiency of patient care.

PATIENT WAIT TIME

The patient is the center of any healthcare organization's focus, and providing immediate access is critical for best outcomes and patient retention. Every aspect of the patient experience, especially confidence in the care provider and perceived quality of care, correlates negatively with longer wait times. Clifford Bleustein and colleagues (2014) found that the decrease in satisfaction scores is associated with an increase in waiting time. Satisfaction scores are more sensitive to exam room waiting times than they are to waiting room wait times.

A survey conducted by Software Advice found that the average wait time in clinician practices was 20 minutes (Hedges 2019). Wait times in hospital-owned physician practices were 17 minutes. More than 50 percent of the physicians surveyed indicated that their patients encountered wait times longer than 20 minutes "often," and 61 percent of physicians have heard negative feedback from their patients regarding wait times. While 63 percent of the physicians in the sample believed wait times had "no impact" or "minimal impact" on their ability to retain patients, 26 percent of patients indicated that they have switched doctors because of long wait times. Further, 64 percent of the physicians surveyed agreed that patient arrival times (e.g., patients arriving later than their scheduled appointment time) are usually the biggest reason they run behind schedule. Notably, 88 percent of the patients in the survey indicated that being told in advance what the wait time will be could help reduce frustration. The Ninth Annual Vitals Wait Time Report found that 36 percent of the patient surveyed said they have left appointments because their wait time became too burdensome (Larson 2018).

SHORTENING WAIT TIMES

The Institute for Healthcare Improvement has offered six principles for reducing wait times (Institute for Healthcare Improvement 2019):

- Recognizing that it is the supply variation of doctors that causes the waiting times and rebalancing the demand and supply for appointments by scheduling patients when demand is predictably lower (early mornings or late in the week)
- Recalibrating the system after eliminating the backlog
- Applying a queuing approach to reducing the number of appointment types; this may free schedulers and receptionists from trying to figure out what patients want
- Creating contingency plans to handle predicted demand and supply variation
- Influencing the demand continuity; development of service agreements between primary care and specialty care to help clarify the referral process
- Managing the rate limiting (i.e., the flow of patients) by proactively establishing which patients are assigned to which physicians in the practice and by redirecting work that can be done by someone else to physician assistants and nurse practitioners

Other ideas include teaching patients to self-triage to ensure they do not seek unnecessarily high-level care. Some health plans increase patients' copayments for nonurgent ED visits (Daly 2017). Health facilities are also enforcing a late arrivals policy and charging patients for short notice cancellations or no-shows. The use of automatic reminders leading up to the appointment helps reduce scheduling errors. Health facilities should review these options with patients and inform patients about no-show or late arrival policies.

Becker's Hospital Review lists the following suggestions to reduce patient wait times (Zimmerman 2016):

- Identify a physician leader who can champion policies designed to monitor wait times and streamline practice scheduling
- Review the average wait time for subsequent available appointments and the frequency of cancellations or no-shows; avoid the first and last appointments (which are not reliable metrics because they are in relatively higher demand)
- Examine providers' schedules to determine whether physician–patient interaction time is optimal
- Administer the benefits verification process and any authorizations prior to each appointment or have patients fill out paperwork ahead of their visit
- Remove phones from the greeting desk to allow front desk employees to maintain eye contact with patients. Instead, assign designated employees to monitor phones in a separate office.

CONVENIENCE

Stryker Performance Solutions, a strategic solutions marketing company at which Dr. Richard Conn serves as medical director, designs "destination center" programs that offer exceptional patient experiences (*Becker's Hospital Review* 2014). These programs improve an organization's transparency, cultivate a strong brand and culture, emphasize leadership, and help organizations create and track benchmarks. Ultimately, destination centers can increase patient volume, improve clinical quality and patient satisfaction, and increase profitability.

DEMAND FOR PHYSICIANS

Demand for physicians continues to grow faster than supply. For all specialties, the retirement decisions of practicing doctors will have

What Happens When I Call for a Same-Day Appointment?

When you call 216.444.CARE or 888.223.CARE, we search across 23 Cleveland Clinic locations throughout Northeast Ohio for an appointment that suits your needs. If you call *before* noon, we will offer you a same-day appointment and if you call *after* noon, we'll offer you an appointment for the next day.

Here is what to expect:

1. We will ask you for basic identifying information, such as address, phone number and insurance carrier.
2. Next, we will ask you a series of questions about your symptoms to help find the most appropriate doctor to treat you. In most cases, we'll be able to schedule the appointment with this information.
3. If you have a complex or chronic medical condition, your call may be triaged by a nurse. This ensures that your physician will receive adequate medical records and other information necessary to give you the best care.

Regardless of the reason for your call, the majority of patients will have an appointment when they hang up with our schedulers.

—Cleveland Clinic (2019)

the greatest effect on future physician supply. More than one-third of all active physicians will be 65 or older by 2030. By that year, the physician shortage will exceed 100,000 (Mann 2017). For primary care, the estimated shortfall will range between 14,800 and 49,300 physicians. Non–primary care specialties—including medical, surgical, and others—are expected to experience a shortfall of 33,800 to 72,700 non–primary care physicians. The projected increase in demand for surgeons will be offset by a small growth in the supply of surgeons, resulting in a shortage of 19,800–29,000 by 2030. For other specialties—emergency medicine, anesthesiology, radiology, neurology, and psychiatry, among others—the projected shortage by 2030 will be between 18,600 and 31,800.

The primary factors driving demand are population growth and an increase in the number of older Americans. Between 2016 and 2030, the US population is projected to increase by about 11 percent, from 324 million to 359 million. The population younger than 18 is estimated to grow by only 3 percent, while the population of people older than 65 is projected to grow by 50 percent. The number of individuals who are more than 75 years old will grow by 73 percent during the same period.

Because seniors have a much higher per capita consumption of healthcare, the demand for physicians—especially specialty physicians—is expected to increase at a much higher rate. This makes the projected shortage especially troubling given that older patients visit health providers, mostly in specialty care, two to three times more often as younger patients do (Dall et al. 2018).

Benchmarks exist on the national level, and they allow a health system's planners to determine whether the area can support more doctors in this specialty. For example, the consulting firm Solucient has prepared a chart of expected patient demand for physicians in various specialty groups, which is used to evaluate the market saturation in regions of the United States (see exhibit 12.1). Demand is expressed as the ratio of the number of full-time-equivalent (FTE) physicians needed to serve 100,000 people in a given geographic area.

Exhibit 12.1: Physician FTE Demand Projections per 100,000 Population, United States

Physician Specialty	FTE Demand per 100,000 Population				
	Nation	Midwest	Northeast	South	West
Primary care					
General and family medicine	22.53	27.85	18.98	22.48	20.20
Internal medicine	19.01	14.22	21.83	20.05	19.86
Pediatrics general	13.90	11.91	17.09	12.70	15.20
Medical specialties					
Allergy/immunology	1.72	1.13	1.54	1.98	2.02
Cardiology	4.22	3.55	6.77	3.44	3.91
Dermatology	3.13	2.30	3.97	3.18	3.19
Gastroenterology	3.50	1.64	3.53	4.40	3.95
Hematology/ oncology	1.08	1.28	0.92	1.03	1.08
Nephrology	0.73	0.37	0.30	0.98	1.10
Neurology	1.79	0.92	1.75	2.10	2.21
Physical medicine and rehabilitation	1.44	1.37	1.95	1.11	1.64
Psychiatry	5.73	4.79	8.86	4.45	6.04
Pulmonary	1.30	0.94	1.59	1.82	0.54
Rheumatology	1.33	1.00	1.46	1.53	1.20
Other medical specialties	2.01	2.83	3.08	0.64	2.51
Surgical specialties					
General surgery	6.01	6.68	5.82	6.42	4.79
Obstetrics and gynecology	10.17	9.10	10.20	11.81	8.57
Ophthalmology	4.71	3.98	5.77	4.52	4.83

(continued)

Orthopedic surgery	6.12	4.46	7.50	5.77	7.18
Otolaryngology	2.84	3.22	2.46	2.86	2.72
Plastic surgery	2.22	1.72	3.06	2.28	1.95
Urology	2.86	2.52	3.54	2.95	2.45
Other surgical specialties	2.20	2.86	2.60	1.52	2.29
Pediatric subspecialties					
Pediatric cardiology	0.20	0.13	0.15	0.26	0.22
Pediatric neurology	0.12	0.14	0.07	0.10	0.18
Pediatric psychiatry	0.59	0.52	0.84	0.59	0.45
Other pediatric subspecialties	0.89	0.89	0.81	0.79	1.10
Emergency department	12.34	12.30	12.65	13.07	10.98
Grand total all specialties	**134.69**	**124.62**	**149.10**	**134.83**	**132.36**

Source: Adapted from Bureau of Health Professions (2008).

MARKETING COMMUNICATION AND CO-BRANDING

Patient empowerment and social media create little margin for error in an external media budget that is expected to produce a measurable return on investment, so targeted marketing and consistency in digital and print media are critical. From websites and social media tools to patient portals and mobile apps for marketing, advertising, and public relations, hospitals can get consumers' attention through targeted zip code marketing, websites, social media posts, and virtual physician visits. Advertising in newspapers and on radio, television, and billboards helps to target audiences that need to know that the hospital or medical group has the solution for their healthcare needs.

Getting the word out about healthcare organizations' technology is also crucial. Robotics such as the Da Vinci Surgical System, a robot used in prostate removal and other surgical procedures, should be included in marketing strategies to increase brand reputation and attract patients.

Enhancing visibility and reputational assets by joining a well-respected brand name or co-brand with 50/50 parity or by creating a new logo for the partnership can be integrated with a marketing strategy. For example, Unity Health joined the Mayo Clinic Care Network in May 2016, pledging to share Mayo Clinic's patient-centered culture and commitment to improving the delivery of healthcare (Unity Health 2019). While Mayo Clinic has other affiliations, this collaboration also allows Mayo to shine as a leading global healthcare network, a win–win strategy.

Another example is the Memorial Sloan Kettering (MSK) Cancer Alliance, which has the overarching goal to improve the lives of cancer patients through dynamic partnerships with local care providers. The MSK Cancer Alliance seeks mutual acceptance of a shared vision and collaboration. Each partnership reflects the uniqueness of its member needs. Components may include the adoption of MSK standards of care, as well as gaining access to the rich portfolio of clinical trials (Memorial Sloan Kettering Cancer Center 2019b).

In 2014, Hartford HealthCare Cancer Institute (HHCCI), which comprises the five cancer programs of Hartford HealthCare's multi-hospital system in Connecticut, became the first member of the MSK Cancer Alliance. It is worth noting that MSK awarded membership to HHCCI only after a thorough analysis of six disease specialties (breast, colorectal, kidney, lung, prostate, and uterine cancer) and 11 disciplines across the institute (Memorial Sloan Kettering Cancer Center 2019a).

Healthcare and Hospital System Co-branding Strategies

Aetna is a good example of a healthcare company that created guidelines and decision trees to determine which branding approach would be optimal for particular situations. To meet its requirements under the Accountable [*sic*] Care Act (ACA), Aetna has entered into a number of hospital partnerships to improve efficiency and affordability, including Banner Health, University Hospitals and Inova, to mention a few.

Aetna created guidelines for how to brand these partnerships, based on what it calls a PADU model—that is, what approach is preferred, acceptable, discouraged or unacceptable. The intent is to optimize the role of the Aetna brand while recognizing the local presence and brand equity of the partner. For example, in localities where the Aetna brand is strong enough to best represent the partnership, it would strive to use a 50/50 linked co-brand with Aetna as the lead (the preferred approach). This is the case with its ACO with University Hospitals.

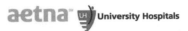

In other situations, where it would be more prudent to emphasize the hospital system since they have more equity and will be more involved with day-to-day operations, the order was reversed (the acceptable approach). This is the case with its ACO with Banner Health.

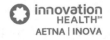

In other partnerships, the decision tree led to a new name (discouraged unless the right criteria are met). This is the case with Innovation Health endorsed by the partners.

⊙ innovation
HEALTH™
AETNA | INOVA

—Thackway McCord (2017)

KEY TAKEAWAYS

- Good strategy links the organization's mission to action, but good strategy also links actions to important organizational goals.
- The planning effort relies on data and information about the external market and internal capabilities, but also on insights and thoughtful study of the business.
- A successful hospital–physician alignment must be more than economic in nature. It must have mutual expectations shared by the hospital and physicians.
- The primary factors driving demand are population growth and an increase in the number of older Americans.
- Benchmarks exist on the national level, and they allow the health system's planners to determine whether the region can support more doctors in this specialty.
- Consider boosting your visibility and reputation through co-branding.

REFERENCES

Allen, M. 2017. "Epidemic of Healthcare Waste: From $1,877 Ear Piercing to ICU Overuse." NPR. Published November 28. www.npr.org/sections/health-shots/2017/11/28/566782829/epidemic-of-health-care-waste-from-1-877-ear-piercing-to-icu-overuse.

Baghai, R., E. H. Levin, and S. Sutaria. 2008. "Service-Line Strategies for US Hospitals." Published July. McKinsey & Company. https://healthcare.mckinsey.com/service-line-strategies-for-us-hospitals.

Becker's Hospital Review. 2014. "5 Tips for Successful Marketing Strategies for Healthcare Organizations." Accessed November 10. www.beckershospitalreview.com/hospital

-management-administration/5-tips-for-successful-marketing
-strategies-for-healthcare-organizations.html.

Belasen, A. R., and A. T. Belasen. 2018. "Doctor-Patient Communication: A Review and a Rationale for Using an Assessment
Framework." *Journal of Healthcare Organization and Management* 32 (7): 891–907.

Belasen, A., B. Eisenberg, and J. Huppertz. 2015. *Mastering Leadership: A Vital Resource for Healthcare Organizations*. Burlington,
MA: Jones & Bartlett Learning.

Bleustein, C., D. B. Rothschild, A. Valen, E. Valatis, L. Schweitzer,
and R. Jones. 2014. "Wait Times, Patient Satisfaction Scores,
and the Perception of Care." *American Journal of Managed Care*
20 (5): 393–400.

Bureau of Health Professions. 2008. *The Physician Workforce: Projections and Research into Current Issues Affecting Supply and
Demand.* US Department of Health and Human Services. Published December. https://bhw.hrsa.gov/sites/default/files/
bhw/nchwa/projections/physiciansupplyissues.pdf.

Byers, J. 2018. "More Than Half of US Physicians Burned
Out, New Study Finds." *Healthcare Dive*. Published January 18. www.healthcaredive.com/news/physician-burnout
-depression-2018/514970.

Cleveland Clinic. 2019. "Same-Day Appointments." Accessed
March 11. https://my.clevelandclinic.org/patients/information/
same-day-appointments.

Dall, T., T. West, R. Chakrabarti, R. Reynolds, and W. Iacobucci.
2018. "The Complexities of Physician Supply and Demand: Projections from 2016 to 2030." Association of American Medical
Colleges. Published March. https://aamc-black.global.ssl.fastly
.net/production/media/filer_public/85/d7/85d7b689-f417-
4ef0-97fb-ecc129836829/aamc_2018_workforce_projections_
update_april_11_2018.pdf.

Daly, R. 2017. "No-Pay Policy for Non-Emergent ED Use Spreading." Healthcare Financial Management Association. Published June 7. www.hfma.org/EDUse.

Hedges, L. 2019. "Practices Must Reduce Wait Times—Here's How." Software Advice. Accessed March 11. www.software advice.com/resources/reducing-patient-wait-times.

Institute for Healthcare Improvement. 2019. "Shortening Wait Times: Six Principles for Improved Access." Accessed March 11. www.ihi.org/resources/Pages/ImprovementStories/Shortening WaitingTimesSixPrinciplesforImprovedAccess.aspx.

Kaplan. 2019. "Predicting Top Medical Specialties for 2019." Accessed March 11. www.kaptest.com/study/mcat/predicting -top-medical-specialties-for-2018/.

Larson, G. 2018. "9th Annual Vitals Wait Time Report Released." Vitals. Published March 22. www.vitals.com/about/posts/ press-center/press-releases/9th-annual-vitals-wait-time-report -released.

Lovelace, B., Jr. 2018. "Hospital Profitability Sinks to Levels Not Seen Since the Financial Crisis: Moody's." CNBC. Published April 24. www.cnbc.com/2018/04/24/hospital-profitability -sinks-to-levels-not-seen-since-financial-crisis.html.

Mann, S. 2017. "Research Shows Shortage of More Than 100,000 Doctors by 2020." *AAMC News*. Published March 14. https:// news.aamc.org/medical-education/article/new-aamc-research -reaffirms-looming-physician-shor.

Memorial Sloan Kettering Cancer Center. 2019a. "MSK Cancer Alliance." Accessed March 11. www.mskcc.org/about/ innovative-collaborations/msk-alliance.

———. 2019b. "MSK Cancer Alliance Members." Accessed March 11. www.mskcc.org/about/innovative-collaborations/ msk-alliance/members.

National Committee for Quality Assurance. 2012. *HEDIS 2013: Healthcare Effectiveness Data and Information Set: Vol. 1*. Washington, DC: National Committee for Quality Assurance.

Thackway McCord. 2017. "Healthcare and Hospital System Co-branding Strategies." Published November 10. www.thackway mccord.com/blog/healthcare-hospital-system-co-branding -strategies.

Transparency Market Research. 2019. "Hybrid Operating Room Market to Attain a Valuation of US$828.1 Billion by 2022; Inclusion of Robot-Assisted Surgeries Plays Crucial Role in Expanding the Market, Says TMR." Published February 14. www.prnewswire.com/news-releases/hybrid-operating-room -market-to-attain-a-valuation-of-us828-1-billion-by-2022 -inclusion-of-robot-assisted-surgeries-plays-crucial-role-in -expanding-the-market-says-tmr-300795719.html.

Unity Health. 2019. "Unity Health and Mayo Clinic: Working Together. Working for You." Accessed March 11. https://unity -health.org/mayo.

US Food and Drug Administration. 2017. "Appropriate Use." Updated December 2. www.fda.gov/radiation-emitting products/radiationsafety/radiationdosereduction/ucm299354 .htm.

Zimmerman, B. 2016. "5 Ways to Reduce Patient Wait Times." *Becker's Hospital Review*. Published August 29. www.beckers hospitalreview.com/patient-flow/5-ways-to-reduce-patient-wait -times.html.

CHAPTER 13

Positive Outcomes

INTRODUCTION

Dyad leaders succeed by focusing on broad directional goals while also analyzing and evaluating how the health system will achieve those goals. They also pay attention to relational goals (e.g., those addressed in the role of patient advocate) while simultaneously addressing functional goals (e.g., those addressed in the role of clinical integration champion).

When managers overemphasize one set of values (or play certain roles excessively without considering the other roles), the organization may become dysfunctional. We often see this occurring among leaders, inside and outside healthcare, who focus almost exclusively on broad vision and directional goals, leaving the hard work of implementation to others (Rumelt 2011).

We also see it when leaders overly focus on the day-to-day routine of operations, failing to discern external events that will bring rapid and significant change to the environment. Such a single-minded pursuit of one set of goals without paying needed attention to the other values or roles creates suboptimization. As exhibit 13.1 illustrates, this is where the overlapping roles and complementary skills of the dyad are useful for balancing directional with functional goals.

Any effort to initiate strategic and operational improvements, align structure with strategy, and link performance indicators with measurable goals should include physician leaders and hospital administrators. Physician leaders send strong signals to external stakeholders that they understand both the clinical and administrative sides of the business; therefore, their inclusion in executive dyads and top leadership roles is essential for the success of the clinically integrated network.

A HOSPITAL LOOKS TO ITS OWN HEALTH: EASTERN MAINE MEDICAL CENTER

The following sections, taken from FTI Consulting's case study, details the history of Eastern Maine Medical Center (EMMC) as

Exhibit 13.1: Dyad Leadership and the Value Strategist's Domain of Operation

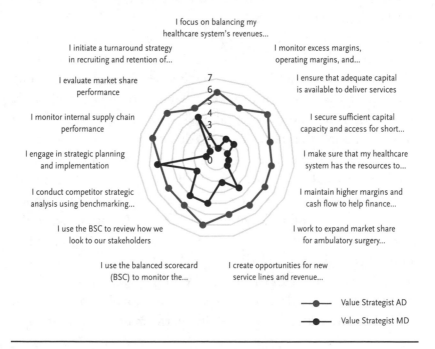

it attempted to improve its financial standing. Supported by FTI Consulting,[1] EMMC quickly identified and implemented labor expense improvements, trained managers and internal consultants on implemented tools, and monitored systems, policies, and procedures to ensure sustained improvement. In addition, FTI Consulting worked with EMMC's physicians and executives to develop and evolve into a patient centered, physician-led, professionally managed medical group.

Background

EMMC serves as the flagship institution for Eastern Maine Health System's (EMHS) network of eight hospitals, the second largest healthcare system in Maine. The 411-bed facility identified the need to improve financial performance ahead of opening their $247 million campus expansion project. EMMC had established a $32 million performance improvement goal for 2014, but six months into the fiscal year, the hospital was falling behind. Instead of achieving a budgeted operating income of $8.8 million, the hospital was operating at a loss of $6.7 million (FTI Consulting 2017).

That kind of loss was a new experience for EMMC. The hospital needed enhanced labor productivity and monitoring, as well as vacancy management procedures to improve and control labor costs. To help address these challenges, EMMC reached out to FTI Consulting.

Productivity Targets That Work

Labor expense management represents a key focus for improved fiscal strength for healthcare organizations.

At EMMC, FTI Consulting performed comprehensive assessments of labor efficiencies and premium pay practices, along with a thorough review of how the hospital compared to its peers. FTI identified specific opportunities for productivity improvement and the steps necessary to realize them, and it worked with leaders at EMMC to achieve and sustain those improvements.

FTI consultants worked with EMMC executives to improve vacancy management by establishing defined criteria for approving requests to fill staff openings (as well as to determine whether each should be a full-time, part-time, or per diem position). FTI also worked with departmental leaders to improve staffing processes and increase the availability of flexible staffing (FTI Consulting 2017).

FTI Consulting also identified opportunities to improve monitoring in an effort to reduce usage of contract labor and "sitters"—aides who stay with patients in certain situations—by instituting evidence-based criteria to better identify patient needs. They

guided the hospital in implementing Labor Analytics, a web-based solution that delivers online access to labor management through advanced visualizations and follow-up reports detailing performance relative to productivity targets. Targets were developed, starting with a national database of peer organizations, along with appropriate normalizations to ensure comparability of the data (FTI Consulting 2017).

FTI experts worked closely with service managers and internal consultants from EMMC's organizational effectiveness group (OEG) to consider operating characteristics at EMMC (e.g., size and geography of services) in designing customized targets. Working with the OEG staff was considered a critical component of ensuring the sustainability of improved policies, procedures, and expenses.

EMHS' seven additional hospitals, as well as its reference lab, have all implemented Labor Analytics. A systemwide productivity committee is now responsible for the centralized governance that allows consistency, comparison, and internal benchmarking (FTI Consulting 2017).

FTI Consulting Role: Establish a High-Performing Medical Group

FTI consultants worked with EMMC executives to develop a high-performing medical group by involving physician leaders and engaging them in strategic and operational improvements. Together, FTI, executives, and physician leaders identified a structure that expanded the number of physicians engaged through the development of a Medical Group Oversight Committee. Later, they developed the Physician Leadership Council, which is made up of four elected physicians, the chief medical officer, the chief financial officer, and the chief administrative officer (CAO). FTI had recommended and recruited a CAO to lead the early stages of development (George 2018).

> FTI Consulting conducted a comprehensive assessment that evaluated critical drivers of financial and operational performance. We then compared the medical group to industry benchmarks and FTI performance measures, conducted practice site visits, and interviewed key stakeholders—to validate what the data was telling us and to better understand both operational and cultural challenges to lasting improvement. The assessment and recommendations included a detailed management action plan and timeline.
>
> FTI worked with the medical group's leadership to develop a structure of working groups to address operational deficiencies and performance opportunities by engaging physician and practice leaders in five Work Streams—Practice

Operations, Patient Access and Referral Management, Revenue Cycle, Practice Performance, and Service Strategy. These work streams meet at least monthly to address gaps in processes and have led to the identification of Medical Group standards that are being implemented across the medical group (FTI Consulting 2017).

The consultants from FTI guided the medical group in implementing Provider Analytics, a web-based solution that provides interactive analytics and insight and delivers monthly reports detailing performance outcomes against productivity, patient access measures, and overall financial measures (George 2018).

In addition to the reduction of labor costs and the formation of a medical group, EMMC engaged FTI to help drive operational improvement in the areas of perioperative care, clinical throughput and length of stay, and financial metrics.

Perioperative Care

The consultants worked with EMMC in an effort to improve operating room efficiency, throughput, and access for patients. EMMC and FTI were successful in leveraging the existing governance to drive change through the development of policies and procedures, improved training, and infrastructure support and development. FTI and the perioperative leadership used metric-driven decision-making to deploy policies related to patient access, scheduling, and block management (George 2018).

Hospitalists, Clinical Throughput, and Length of Stay

FTI consultants provided change management and consulting services aimed at identifying priorities for improving program performance, including outcomes, communication and collaboration across disciplines, and engagement of hospitalist physicians. They also provided coaching and mentoring for the hospitalist leadership. They developed and facilitated a multi-stakeholder working group focused on improving quality of care satisfaction, efficiency, and throughput. As a result, individual hospitalists reported improved morale and engagement with respect to the strategic goals of the hospital, and hospital leadership uniformly expressed the more effective alignment with the hospitalist program (George 2018).

Upgrading patient throughput was a specific clinical area of focus for the team. In order to improve, the consultants helped to redesign the role of case management, refocusing on care coordination and proactive discharge planning. They also instituted multidisciplinary rounds (MDRs) on all nursing units, attended by key disciplines including hospitalists, pharmacy, nursing, and case management and established anticipated discharge dates for all patients with plans to meet the goals. MDRs were supported by the development of geographic rounding for hospitalists and improved handoffs from emergency medicine physicians to hospitalists (George 2018).

Financial Metrics

> The annualized financial impact of hospital labor and productivity improvements from October 2014 through January 2015 showed labor expense reductions of approximately $8.2 million (compared to an estimate of $6.8 million). The January 2015 operating margin for EMMC was approximately $10 million. In the same period the previous year, the hospital incurred a $6 million operating loss (FTI Consulting 2017).

Testimonials

James A. Raczek, MD, FAAFP, senior vice president and chief medical officer for EMMC, provided client leadership for the clinical and medical group engagements. He believes that FTI provided the right blend of expertise and support necessary to achieve operational and financial improvement.

FTI provided key support at a critical time to help us drive the transformation of our Medical Group, collaborating with us to establish a governance structure, providing interim CAO support and the formation of a Leadership Council consisting of peer-elected physician members. With FTI's assistance we have engaged physician and nonphysician providers to achieve improved operational and financial performance and continue to further enhance our vision of being a patient-centered, physician led, and professionally managed Medical Group (FTI Consulting 2017).

Deborah Sanford, RN, a vice president and chief nursing officer who helped to lead the engagement from the system-steering committee before accepting her current role, believes that working collaboratively with FTI was extremely beneficial to achieving financial sustainability.

They assisted us in the coaching and mentoring of our front line and middle managers to support the changes we needed. Going on two years later we continue to sustain the gains we initially made and continue to utilize benchmarking and leadership best practices to allow for further improvements.

KEY TAKEAWAYS

- As the clinically integrated network is increasingly evolving into a complex system, the focal point of the healthcare sector is shifting away from hospitals. Dyad leaders must focus on an overarching visions and broader clinical alignment goals.
- In the role of value strategist, the dyad has to contain the managerial, leadership, and communication skills to handle key internal and external interfaces.

- The cycle of continuous improvement must include both physicians and administrators.
- Engaging external consultants who provide interactive analytics, insights, and reports can help achieve positive outcomes in patient access, practice performance, practice operations, service strategy, and revenue cycle and referral management.

NOTE

1. FTI Consulting, Inc, is an independent global business advisory firm dedicated to helping organizations manage change and mitigate risk: financial, legal, operational, political and regulatory, reputational, and transactional. FTI Consulting professionals, located in all major business centers throughout the world, work closely with clients to anticipate, illuminate, and overcome complex business challenges and opportunities. www.fticonsulting.com.

REFERENCES

FTI Consulting. 2017. *A Hospital Looks to Its Own Health*. Accessed April 3, 2019. www.fticonsulting.com/~/media/Files/us-files/insights/case-studies/hospital-looks-to-its-own-health.pdf.

George, C. 2018. Correspondence with author.

Rumelt, R. 2011. "The Perils of Bad Strategy. *McKinsey Quarterly*. Published June. www.mckinsey.com/business-functions/strategy-and-corporate-finance/our-insights/the-perils-of-bad-strategy.

PART IV

Role: Clinical Integration Champion

Exhibit 4: Clinical Integration Champion

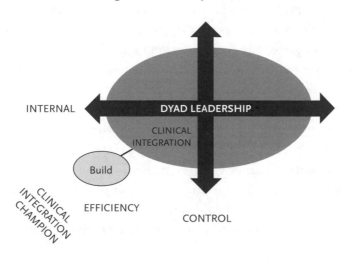

With healthcare systems shifting away from encounter-based reimbursement toward new incentives that reward coordination of care and population health management, many hospitals are also consolidating into clinically integrated networks to optimize processes, improve patient care, and reduce operating costs. The American Hospital Association (2010) describes clinical integration as "the means to facilitate the coordination of patient care across conditions, providers, settings, and time in order to achieve care that is safe, timely, effective, efficient, equitable, and patient-focused."

Despite efforts by the Affordable Care Act and the Centers for Medicare & Medicaid Services to expand coverage, boost the effectiveness and efficiency of processes and outcomes, and increase the quality of care, many hospitals still cannot ensure true clinical integration because they are locked in silos with limited coordination across the continuum of care.

With limited coordination across multiple specialty groups or settings, patients are more likely to receive duplicate diagnostic tests, have adverse prescription drug interactions, and get conflicting care plans. The shift to value-based payment methods, on the other hand, transfers financial risk to physicians and hospitals, changes the fabric of the patient experience, and creates incentives for clinical integration across the continuum of care.

Chapter 14 introduces clinically integrated networks in the context of meeting the goals of the Triple Aim. Chapter 15 links clinical integration with collaborative leadership and the opportunity to coordinate and manage quality across the continuum of care. Chapter 16 covers dyad leadership that focuses on a culture of safety and reliability. Chapter 17 covers the importance of teamwork and interfunctional collaboration. When clinical and nonclinical staff collaborate effectively, healthcare teams can improve patient outcomes, prevent medical errors, improve efficiency, and increase patient satisfaction.

REFERENCE

American Hospital Association. 2010. "Clinical Integration—The Key to Real Reform." *Trendwatch*. Published February. www .aha.org/research/reports/tw/10feb-clinicinteg.pdf.

CHAPTER 14

The Context for the Dyad Clinical Integration Champion

INTRODUCTION

Clinical integration creates meaningful cross-specialty service lines that support the Triple Aim:

1. Improving the patient experience of care (including quality and satisfaction)
2. Improving the health of populations
3. Reducing the per capita cost of healthcare

To change current behaviors and expectations, dyad leaders engage in activities and roles that reach beyond the clinical setting and incorporate the interests and goals of patients, communities, and public health systems.

These leaders focus on delivery systems based on an integrated strategy through accountable care organizations (ACOs), bundled payments, and financing. They employ innovative models of primary care, including patient-centered medical homes, and create disincentives for avoidable events, including hospital readmission. They prioritize meaningful use of electronic health records to improve quality, safety, and efficiency and to reduce health disparities. Clinical integration within the scope of the Triple Aim is the focus of this chapter.

CLINICAL INTEGRATION

Hospitals that can integrate innovation and safety in operations, planning and coordination, and adaptability and reliability will have a more successful outcome in meeting the goals of the Triple Aim.

The ability of health systems to expand the boundaries of population health to encompass the larger community depends on adequate resources and capabilities, appropriate size and market share, and a culture of teamwork and collaboration. Meeting these goals requires

- organizing around the needs of patients rather than physicians,
- partnerships among providers and payers,
- integrated information technology capabilities,
- interprofessional collaboration,
- a shift away from a fee-for-service structure to a value-based structure,
- bundled payment,
- capitation,
- increased financial risk sharing for the populations served, and
- shared accountability for population health outcomes.

There is a wide range of approaches and strategies for achieving successful clinical integration. For example, a collaborative setting—one that includes physicians, hospitals, and post-acute care providers aligned around shared risk and around protocols to improve quality and reduce the cost of care—helps members to keep their independence and maintain control over their practices or institutions, a feature that is often lost in a full merger. Autonomy and discretion empower physicians to determine choices based on personal needs, goals, and career ambitions.

REDUCING HOSPITAL READMISSIONS

Reducing hospital readmissions is a current priority for the health-care system. While no single strategy has a sustainable effect in preventing rehospitalization, timely follow-up with patients at discharge has always been a key success factor in reducing readmission rates. Hudali, Robinson, and Bhattarai (2017) have confirmed that patients who received follow-up calls from nurses and who also attended the discharge consultation had significantly lower 30-day readmission rates (3.8 percent, compared to 11.7 for people who did neither). A Cox regression analysis showed that the transition of care (TOC) clinic attendance had a significant negative predication for readmission: a hazard ratio of 0.186, a 95 percent confidence interval 0.038–0.898, and a p value equal to 0.038. (A small p value or calculated probability, typically less than or equal to 0.05, indicates strong evidence against the null hypothesis—i.e., patients without follow-up calls and TOC—so it is rejected).

Bradley and colleagues (2013) analyzed cross-sectional data from a 2010–2011 online survey of 585 hospitals in a national quality initiative to reduce heart failure readmissions. The researchers have identified six strategies that hospitals could deploy to reduce readmissions. These strategies are consistent with the structure of clinical integration, including the following:

1. Partnering with community physicians and physician groups
2. Collaborating with local facilities to develop consistent readmission reduction strategies
3. Assigning nurses to manage medication reconciliation
4. Scheduling follow-up appointments for patients prior to discharge

5. Assigning staff to follow up with patients on postdischarge test results that return after the patient is discharged

6. Having a process in place to send all discharge papers or electronic summaries directly to the patient's primary physician

CLINICALLY INTEGRATED NETWORKS MEET FEDERAL TRADE COMMISSION REQUIREMENTS

The term *clinical integration* describes networks with a range of engagement strategies among members, extending from loose affiliations to mergers. These networks could form out of a vague collaboration among longtime rivals, becoming joint ventures with contractual agreements. They could also arise from mergers that bring hospitals and physicians under single ownership, leaving the network open to scrutiny for possible anticompetitive practices under antitrust law.

Clinical Integration in Healthcare: A Check-Up

Clinical integration is a term used to describe certain types of collaborations among otherwise independent healthcare providers to improve quality and contain costs. The 1996 joint FTC [Federal Trade Commission]/Department of Justice Statements of Antitrust Enforcement Policy in Health Care expressly recognizes the relevance of such integration to the antitrust analysis of healthcare provider networks that seek to collectively negotiate contracts with payers on behalf of their members.

—Federal Trade Commission (2008)

Under the Department of Justice and the FTC, the term *clinically integrated network* (CIN) refers to a specific legal arrangement that allows competing caregivers to contract with payers jointly. For example, providers may collaborate to manage and coordinate care for Medicare fee-for-service beneficiaries through an ACO.

Competition in healthcare markets benefits consumers because it helps contain costs, improve quality, and encourage innovation. The FTC's job as a law enforcer is to stop firms from engaging in anticompetitive conduct that harms consumers.

Clinical integration is legally acceptable if the CIN goal is to improve patient care, not simply to bargain for better rates (Gosfield and Reinertsen 2010). The CIN needs to have a legal structure for contracting with payers and, in turn, paying physicians based on outcomes, not referrals. To be acceptable under FTC standards, it must be an independently governed entity with the objective of improving population health through coordinated programs and interventions. The innate structure of a CIN is aimed at optimizing processes and approaches that yield the best possible outcomes for patients.

The FTC enforces the antitrust laws in healthcare markets to prevent anticompetitive conduct that would deprive consumers of the benefits of competition. The agency also provides guidance to participants in the healthcare market (US Department of Justice and FTC 1996). Antitrust enforcement helps ensure potentially more efficient ways of delivering and financing healthcare while preventing accumulations of market power that harm competition (Canterman 2016).

CLINICALLY INTEGRATED NETWORK

Formally, a CIN can be a physician–hospital organization, an independent practice association, or the subsidiary of a health system, but it must have physician leadership embedded into the governance

The Benefits of a Clinically Integrated Network

Successful CINs operate on a pluralistic approach—multiple components must exist and work together for the organization to flourish. Those components, whether it be individual physicians working side by side or physicians and hospitals coming together, must "operate in a dyad."

—Dr. Ninfa Saunders, quoted by
Alyssa Rege (2016)

model (the dyad helps meet this objective). Networks must have four components to be considered clinically integrated:

1. Physician leadership and commitment
2. Development and implementation of clinical practice guidelines to improve performance
3. Development of infrastructure and technology
4. Sound financial incentives for achieving goals

Successful clinical integration depends on creating appropriate expectations and incentives for physicians, effective implementation of IT infrastructure and tools, and ongoing development of physician leadership capacity. All CIN members must formally commit to complying with clinical guidelines and working on performance improvement activities. Data sharing and performance monitoring are required. The CIN must demonstrate that it is improving value, not just using its size to fix prices with the effect of increasing the cost of physician services and medical insurance for patients (FTC 1998).

Case Studies in Clinical Integration

In Michigan, Together Health Network (THN) has emerged as a "super CIN" composed of nine local CINs that cover the state. THN was formed in 2014 by two large health systems, Ascension and Trinity Health. The University of Michigan Health System joined as an equity partner and quaternary care provider this year.

The network includes more than 5,000 physicians and 29 hospitals, and its leaders estimate that 75 percent of Michigan residents live within 20 minutes of a THN provider. THN's vision is to be the preferred partner of anyone—patients, physicians, or payers—looking for care models that deliver on the so-called Quadruple Aim: better care for individual patients, better population health, lower healthcare costs, and better experiences for healthcare providers.

[. . .]

. . . "We are striving for more clinical integration, and that is why we are spending the time to understand where folks are currently and where we have the opportunity to integrate our clinical informatics systems, our network analytic systems, and our performance improvement processes," [says Scott Eathorne, MD, president and CEO of THN.]

Eventually, THN will implement a dashboard that supports performance improvement throughout the super CIN.

"We are working to establish a common care model by which we work with each of the groups to decrease variation in the care that is provided," he says. "That will be largely managed at the local level."

—Lola Butcher (2016)

KEY TAKEAWAYS

- Dyad leaders engage in activities and roles that reach beyond the clinical setting and incorporate the interests and goals of patients, communities, and public health systems.
- Timely follow-up with patients at discharge has always been a key success factor in reducing readmission rates.
- Clinical integration is legally acceptable if the CIN goal is to improve patient care, not simply to bargain for better rates.
- Successful clinical integration depends on creating appropriate expectations and incentives for physicians, effective implementation of IT infrastructure and tools, and ongoing development of physician leadership capacity.

REFERENCES

Bradley, E. H., L. Curry, L. I. Horwitz, H. Sipsma, Y. Wang, M. N. Walsh, D. Goldmann, N. White, I. L. Pina, and H. M. Krumholz. 2013. "Hospital Strategies Associated with 30-Day Readmission Rates for Patients with Heart Failure." *Circulation: Cardiovascular Quality and Outcomes* 6 (4): 444–50.

Butcher, L. 2016. "Case Studies in Clinical Integration." *Leadership+*. Published November 17. www.hfma.org/Leadership/Archives/2016/Fall/Case_Studies_in_Clinical_Integration.

Canterman, R. S. 2016. "Antitrust and Collaboration in Health Care." American Bar Association. Published March 4. www.americanbar.org/content/dam/aba/administrative/healthlaw/15_canterman.authcheckdam.pdf.

Federal Trade Commission. 2008. "Clinical Integration in Health Care: A Check-Up." Published May 29. www.ftc.gov/news-events/events- calendar/2008/05/clinical-integration-health-care-check.

————. 1998. "Louisiana Group of Doctors to Settle FTC Charges That It Fixed Prices." Published June 19. www.ftc .gov/news-events/press-releases/1998/06/louisiana-group -doctors-settle-ftc-charges-it-fixed-prices.

Gosfield, A. G., and J. L. Reinertsen. 2010. "Achieving Clinical Integration with Highly Engaged Physicians." Institute for Healthcare Improvement. Published December. www.ihi.org/ resources/Pages/Publications/AchievingClinicalIntegration HighlyEngagedPhysicians.aspx.

Hudali, T., R. Robinson, and M. Bhattarai. 2017. "Reducing 30-Day Rehospitalization Rates Using a Transition of Care Clinic Model in a Single Medical Center." *Advances in Medicine.* Published August 2. www.ncbi.nlm.gov/pmc/articles/PMC5558630.

Rege, A. 2016. "The Benefits of a Clinically Integrated Network: 3 Thoughts." *Becker's Hospital Review.* Published September 22. www.beckershospitalreview.com/hospital-transactions -and-valuation/the-benefits-of-a-clinically-integrated-network -3-thoughts.html.

US Department of Justice and Federal Trade Commission. 1996. "Statements of Antitrust Enforcement Policy in Health Care." Published August. www.ftc.gov/sites/default/files /attachments/competition-policy-guidance/statements_of _antitrust_enforcement_policy_in_health_care_august_1996 .pdf.

CHAPTER 15

A Platform for Collaboration

INTRODUCTION

Clinical integration (CI) offers hospitals and physicians the opportunity to coordinate patient interventions, manage quality across the continuum of care, move toward population health management, and pursue true value-based contracting.

The pillars of CI include shared governance (with strong physician leadership) focusing on the transformation of health system culture and the achievement of clinical outcomes—the key drivers toward value-based care (Marino 2012). This requires a mindset of interfunctional collaboration, sharing information, managing utilization, and providing proactive care. Communicating the value of CI, employing innovative care delivery models, and tracking clinical quality outcomes all create incentives for joint accountability, mutual commitment, teamwork, and engagement across the continuum of care.

ALIGNING INCENTIVES

It is essential that clinically integrated networks develop interdisciplinary structures that align goals and incentives. Incentive plans that encourage productivity across the entire spectrum of care must reward physicians' efforts to achieve quality care and reduce cost.

Strategies and decisions must be shared and communicated to the entire organization and resources must be available to support the goal of integration. A key priority is to develop a risk-based cost model that links patient care costs to interventions and quality outcomes. Chief financial officers will need to engage with payers to explore and negotiate risk-based contracts and develop appropriate physician performance incentive programs.

CLINICAL PROGRAMS

Effective coordination between providers and optimization of care transitions will improve patient outcomes and help reduce costs. They will do so by eliminating redundant testing and providing better management of patient care. Important areas of focus include high-risk patients (e.g., patients with diabetes who also have comorbidities such as hypertension or heart failure), cost-control opportunities (e.g., generic drugs, review of magnetic resonance imaging usage), and prevention programs (e.g., smoking cessation and depression screening).

Developing appropriate clinical performance measures is imperative. For example, an asthma care program could track asthma control rates, screening frequency, and currency of asthma action plans. The program could also track cost measures such as drug expenses, physician visits, and emergency department visits.

Clinical programs should also develop care plans that define care protocols for various conditions. Dyad leaders can use process mapping to create care pathways that encompass ambulatory, inpatient, post-acute, and home health interventions. Healthcare process mapping is an important form of clinical audit that examines the patient experience from the patient's perspective to identify problems and suggest improvements.

Creating Value Through Process Mapping

The largest health system in Illinois, Advocate [Health Care], comprises over 250 sites of care, including 12 acute-care hospitals. In developing a process map of the Inpatient Stay care segment, we followed these steps:

1. *Identify a care segment that has opportunities for improvement.* Specific areas . . . include identifying non-value-added clinical and administrative tasks. For each task within a care process, we ask ourselves, "Is this something that a lower-cost resource could be doing, instead of the high-cost alternative?" . . .
2. *Develop a first draft of a care segment process map by interviewing experts—that is, the people involved in the process.* . . .
3. *Start with Post-it notes, then convert to electronic.* . . . [This] surfaced missing steps, highlighted misunderstandings, and allowed us to refer back to it for improvement opportunities.
4. *Observe the care segment twice to validate the process map.* . . . Repeating the observation can catch variations in practice.
5. *Close the loop with the experts after the observation.* . . . Not only does it highlight opportunities for improvement, and identify non-value-added processes, it idenitifies gaps in processes that that subject matter experts and manager believe are occurring all the time, when in reality there are barriers that may lead these processes to only be occurring 30–50% of the time.

Of course, delivering reliably excellent care across teams, units, and sites takes more than creating a process map. Changes to medical practice, such as adjusting staffing skill mix, require negotiation, engagement, and support from physician champions and key leadership.

—Kevin Little and Mike Barbati, as told to
IHI Multimedia Team (2015)

Proactive medicine is key. The success of CI hinges on the physicians' ability to anticipate and prevent patient problems. To do this, clinicians need to incorporate care gap reports into clinical care and adopt new processes—for example, by assigning a nurse to call patients with high-risk diabetes to ensure hemoglobin A1C is reported according to the defined diabetic clinical treatment protocol.

TECHNOLOGY INFRASTRUCTURE

Investments in technologies that support population health make hospital–physician alignment quite attractive, although the peril of overspending on technology infrastructure and underdelivering on functionality must be closely monitored. The key to avoiding these problems is to invest in an electronic health record (EHR) system that connects ambulatory electronic medical records (of both employed and independent physicians), the hospital's data, pharmacy information systems, and labs. The goal is to create a longitudinal patient record that allows physicians, nurses, and other providers across the care community to track patient care in every setting.

A clinically integrated organization needs to be able to aggregate and analyze clinical data to identify performance gaps and develop improvement plans. The key is to incorporate tools that allow the clinically integrated networks (CIN) to run performance analytics on clinical programs, care settings, provider performance, and cost utilization. CINs should also invest in technologies for connecting patients. Patient electronic engagement—via patient portals and secure messaging—is an important requirement under meaningful use or interoperability programs. In fact, the Centers for Medicare & Medicaid Services distributes incentive payments to healthcare providers that effectively implement EHRs and use them to improve quality of care coordination and patient engagement.

BENEFITS OF CLINICAL INTEGRATION

Regardless of the strategy, when designed and implemented appropriately, CI offers tremendous potentials for efficiencies and improvements in healthcare quality and patient satisfaction. Here are ten benefits to consider when exploring the feasibility of CI and options for achieving it (Marino 2019):

1. *Increase collaboration.* The use of cross-functional teams helps to address gaps in the care continuum and implement a CI program effectively.
2. *Improve efficiency.* CI eliminates non-value-added activities and redundancy, allowing health systems to deliver seamless care.
3. *Integrated systems.* CI programs provide health systems with monitoring and enforcement tools, including financial incentives for participating physicians.
4. *Payer partnerships.* As CI improves the quality of patient care and clinical processes and reduces costs, health systems are able to achieve market differentiation that can serve as a lever for further partnerships.
5. *Improved care management.* The goal is to achieve the best clinical and cost outcomes for both patient and provider. This goal is most successful when case managers are able to work inside and outside of coordinated care.
6. *Integrated continuum of care.* CI care management teams collaborate with adult day care, independent living, assisted living, and skilled nursing facility partners to efficiently assess, document, communicate, and meet patient needs.
7. *Clinical data systems.* An integrated health system must also have an integrated technology platform. Information technology should facilitate communication across the care continuum and provide information that measures service,

performance, quality, and outcomes, at the levels of both individual provider and network.

8. *Patient-centered communication.* Reducing barriers to communication and improving doctor–patient communication to help increase patient satisfaction and retention.

9. *Improved pharmaceutical management.* CI improves pharmaceutical management by identifying gaps in the medication management process and allowing hospitals to take actions to help make patients safer.

10. *Improved community health.* CI emphasizes wellness initiatives such as outreach programs and classes to empower patients to participate actively in their care. This restructuring is not a project with a defined endpoint, but an evolution that requires proactive medicine, continuous improvement, dedicated resources, and the combined strengths of dyad leaders.

KEY TAKEAWAYS

- Changes to medical practice (e.g., adjusting staffing skill mix) require negotiation, engagement, and support from physician champions and influential leaders.
- Incentive plans that encourage productivity across the entire spectrum of care must reward physicians' efforts in achieving quality care and reducing cost.
- A key priority is to develop a risk-based cost model coupled with clinical performance measures that link patient care costs to interventions and quality outcomes.
- Dyad leaders can use process mapping to create care pathways that encompass ambulatory, inpatient, post-acute, and home health interventions.

- Proactive medicine and investment in EHR software that connects ambulatory medical records, pharmacy information systems, and labs help sustain CI efforts.

REFERENCES

IHI Multimedia Team. 2015. "5 Steps for Creating Value Through Process Mapping and Observation." Institute for Healthcare Improvement. Published October 1. www.ihi.org/communities /blogs/5-steps-for-creating-value-through-process-mapping -and-observation.

Marino, D. J. 2019. *The Franchise Model: An Emerging Strategy for Clinical Integration*. Health Directions. Accessed March 18. http://cdn2.hubspot.net/hub/161605/file-418142763-pdf/ Original_HD_Publishing/The_Franchise_Model_An_Emerging _Strategy_for_Clinical_Integration.pdf.

———. 2012. "The 4 Pillars of Clinical Integration: A Flexible Model for Hospital-Physician Collaboration." *Becker's Hospital Review*. Published November 14. www.beckershospitalreview .com/hospital-physician-relationships/the-4-pillars-of-clinical -integration-a-flexible-model-for-hospital-physician-collabor ation.html.

CHAPTER 16

Fitting into a Culture of Safety and Reliability

INTRODUCTION

Creating a culture of interprofessional collaboration and cross-functional synergies requires empowerment and self-management, participative forms of leadership and communication, and the use of motivational strategies that match the needs of employees and the complexity of the task environment.

Effective dyad leaders in integrated health systems unify the mission, clarify the strategic vision for their organizations, employ evidence-based best practices to improve patient quality and safety, and enhance the overall efficiency and effectiveness of the organization. The dyad visibly and consistently supports the narratives of interprofessional collaboration and engages in ongoing dialogue with staff and clinicians during the transition and deployment of care teams. This helps to inspire employees to change their way of thinking about patient care and the culture of the organization, avoid confusion during transitions, and facilitate collaborative behaviors.

PROMOTING A CULTURE OF SAFETY AND RELIABILITY

Health systems with a strong culture of safety use transparent communications to build trust and promote joint accountability. Maintaining a safety culture requires leaders to consistently and visibly initiate and track preventive safety measures. According to the Joint Commission Center for Transforming Healthcare (2017), these measures include

- sufficient support of patient safety event reporting,
- meaningful feedback and positive support to staff who report safety vulnerabilities,
- prioritization and implementation of safety provisions,
- measures to resolve staff and clinician burnout, and
- establishing teamwork and building relationships.

Accountable care organizations need to assess which preventive evidence-based services yield improved health outcomes and a strong return on investment for their patients. This could include clinical preventive services (e.g., mammography, immunizations, smoking cessation) and community preventive services (e.g., fluoridation, lead testing, community screening).

Creating a patient-centered culture of safety requires the approach of a high-reliability organization (HRO). An HRO has a collective mindfulness that transcends specialized areas and empowers staff members to collaborate in identifying possible failures and tackling them in a proactive, timely, and responsible manner. Problem identification and problem resolution are fundamental to becoming an HRO.

The Essential Role of Leadership in Developing a Safety Culture

Leaders can build safety cultures by readily and willingly participating with care team members in initiatives designed to develop and emulate safety culture characteristics. Effective leaders who deliberately engage in strategies and tactics to strengthen their organization's safety culture see safety issues as problems with organizational systems, not their employees, and see adverse events and close calls ("near misses") as providing "information-rich" data for learning and systems improvement. Individuals within the organization respect and are wary of operational hazards, have a collective mindfulness that people and equipment will sometimes fail, defer to expertise rather than hierarchy in decision making, and develop defenses and contingency plans to cope with failures. These concepts stem from the extensive research of James Reason on the psychology of human error. Among Reason's description of the main elements of a safety culture are:

- *Just culture*—people are encouraged, even rewarded, for providing essential safety-related information, but clear lines are drawn between human error and at-risk or reckless behaviors.
- *Reporting culture*—people report their errors and near misses.
- *Learning culture*—the willingness and the competence to draw the right conclusions from safety information systems, and the will to implement major reforms when their need is indicated.

In an organization with a strong safety culture, individuals within the organization treat each other and their patients with dignity and respect.

—The Joint Commission (2017)

Becoming a High Reliability Organization

We are . . . focusing on several principles of reliability science:

- Designing reliable, standardized systems that support staff decisions, opportunities for feedback, ongoing learning, and change
- Learning to be more mindful of decisions and actions using HRO theory . . .
- Improving situational awareness—the concept of reliably identifying at-risk patients, lessening their risk, and escalating risks until the patient is safe
- Managing by prediction and having robust plans in place for the expected and the unexpected
- Looking at human factors—how we relate to the world around us and how learning more about how we work and interact, and designing systems that take human factors into account, can help us better keep patients, families, employees, and visitors safe

In HROs, senior leaders are conducting frequent walk-rounds to reinforce safety behaviors and find and fix critical safety issues. They're also meeting in daily operational briefs where they look back to learn from failures and look forward to predict and lessen risk or harm.

Frontline leaders (for example, unit charge nurses) are rounding with staff every day, giving 5:1 positive to negative feedback, conducting daily huddles, and modeling the expected safety behaviors. HRO leaders manage by anticipation and prediction rather than reaction. Frontline leaders focus on predicting events in the next 24 hours and making real-time adjustments to keep patients, families, employees and visitors safe.

—James M. Anderson Center for
Health Systems Excellence, 2019

HRO IN HEALTHCARE

Applying HRO concepts in a healthcare system begins with dyad leaders at all levels initiating a discourse about how to improve the process of caregiving and its outcomes. HRO hallmarks that should become embedded in the health system include the following (Hines et al. 2008):

- *Sensitivity to operations.* HROs maintain constant awareness on the part of leaders, frontline nurses, patient care attendants, technicians, and support staff of the state of the systems and processes that affect patient care. Having situational awareness is key to noting risks, closing loopholes in processes with potential for patient harm, and taking proactive steps for preventing problems.
- *Reluctance to simplify.* Simple processes are good, but simplistic explanations for why things work or fail are risky. Avoiding overly simple explanations of failure (e.g., unqualified staff, inadequate training, communication failure) is essential in order to underscore the reasons patients are at risk. Ask "why" and "what if" questions, solicit expert advice, and swap the dominant thinking with perspectives from others with diverse experience. Leverage new thinking to get to root causes of problems.
- *Preoccupation with failure.* Examine near misses to avoid reoccurrence and learn from them to reduce potential harm to patients. Attention to detail is crucial. Identifying and fixing problems is everyone's responsibility and is encouraged and supported by leadership.

Michigan Health & Hospital Association Joins the Team

Michigan Is the Second State to Partner with the Joint Commission Center for Transforming Healthcare on a Statewide High Reliability Improvement Effort

The Michigan Health & Hospital Association (MHA) and its member hospitals have established a long-standing reputation for leadership on patient safety and quality improvement. At its Nov. 4, 2015, meeting, the MHA Board of Trustees acted to further that commitment by unanimously supporting a motion for Michigan hospitals to begin the journey to become Highly Reliable Organizations (HROs).

Sam R. Watson, MHA's senior vice president of patient safety and quality and executive director of the MHA Keystone Center, said in a recent interview, "Achieving high reliability in healthcare is the next step in improving Michigan's quality of care, reducing costs and minimizing institutional risk for both patients and providers."

The MHA is the second state in the US to collaborate with the Joint Commission Center for Transforming Healthcare on a statewide HRO improvement effort. "High reliability in healthcare signifies excellent care is consistently delivered, with a commitment to zero preventable harm," Watson added.

Michigan's partnership with the Center for Transforming Healthcare will allow Michigan hospitals to systematically look at and develop strategies to improve organizational effectiveness and efficiency, customer satisfaction, compliance, and organizational culture, while ensuring the best care is provided to every patient, every time.

—Joint Commission Center for Transforming Health Care (2019)

- *Deference to expertise.* Leaders who trust frontline teams and experts also accept their insights and suggestions about risks, and they support decisions with quick follow-up.
- *Resilience.* Leaders and staff need to be trained to respond quickly and effectively to deal with system failures.

THE HOSPITAL SURVEY ON PATIENT SAFETY CULTURE

In 2004, as part of its goal to support a culture of patient safety and quality improvement, the Agency for Healthcare Research and Quality (AHRQ) sponsored the development of the Hospital Survey on Patient Safety Culture for hospitals, nursing homes, ambulatory outpatient medical offices, community pharmacies, and ambulatory surgery centers (AHRQ 2019). The purpose was to assess hospital staff opinions about patient safety issues, medical errors, and event reporting. The survey (see exhibit 16.1) included 42 items that measured 12 areas, or composites, of patient safety culture (Westat et al. 2016). The AHRQ program enables healthcare organizations to use these tools to

- raise staff awareness about patient safety,
- diagnose and assess the current status of patient safety culture,
- identify strengths and areas for patient safety culture improvement,
- examine trends in patient safety culture change over time,
- evaluate the cultural impact of patient safety initiatives and interventions, and
- conduct internal and external comparisons.

Exhibit 16.1: AHRQ Patient Safety Culture Composites and Definitions

Patient Safety Culture Composite	Definition: The extent to which . . .
1. Communication openness	Staff freely speak up if they see something that may negatively affect a patient and feel free to question those with more authority.
2. Feedback and communication about error	Staff are informed about errors that happen, are given feedback about changes implemented, and discuss ways to prevent errors.
3. Frequency of events reported	Mistakes of the following types are reported: (1) mistakes caught and corrected before affecting the patient, (2) mistakes with no potential to harm the patient, and (3) mistakes that could harm the patient but do not.
4. Handoffs and transitions	Important patient care information is transferred across hospital units and during shift changes.
5. Management support for patient safety	Hospital management provides a work climate that promotes patient safety and shows that patient safety is a top priority.
6. Nonpunitive response to error	Staff feel that their mistakes and event reports are not held against them and that mistakes are not kept in their personnel file.
7. Organizational learning— continuous improvement	Mistakes have led to positive changes, and changes are evaluated for effectiveness.
8. Overall perceptions of patient safety	Procedures and systems are good at preventing errors, and there is a lack of patient safety problems.
9. Staffing	There are enough staff to handle the workload, and work hours are appropriate to provide the best care for patients.

(continued)

Exhibit 16.1: AHRQ Patient Safety Culture Composites and Definitions *(continued)*

10. Supervisor/ manager expectations and actions promoting patient safety	Supervisors/managers consider staff suggestions for improving patient safety, praise staff for following patient safety procedures, and do not overlook patient safety problems.
11. Teamwork across units	Hospital units cooperate and coordinate with one another to provide the best care for patients.
12. Teamwork within units	Staff support each other, treat each other with respect, and work together as a team.

Source: Adapted from AHRQ (2018).

As exhibit 16.2 shows, the areas of strength or the composites with the highest average percent positive responses were teamwork in units (82 percent), supervisor or manager expectations and actions promoting patient safety (78 percent), and organizational learning—continuous improvement (73 percent). The areas with potential for improvement or the composites with the lowest average percent positive responses were nonpunitive response to error (45 percent), handoffs and transitions (48 percent), and staffing (54 percent).

The survey also included two questions asking respondents to provide an overall rating on patient safety for their work area or unit and to indicate the number of events they reported over the past 12 months. Event reporting was identified as an area for improvement for most health systems because underreporting of events means potential patient safety problems may not be recognized or identified and therefore may not be addressed. Westat and colleagues noted that on average, 45 percent of respondents in hospitals reported that at least one event has occurred at their hospital. It is likely that they are underreported, as respondents are reluctant to admit to mistakes. In comparison, on average, 76 percent of respondents in hospitals gave their work area or unit a grade of "Excellent" (34 percent) or "Very Good" (42 percent) on patient safety.

Exhibit 16.2: Composite-Level Average Percent Positive Response—2016 Database Hospitals

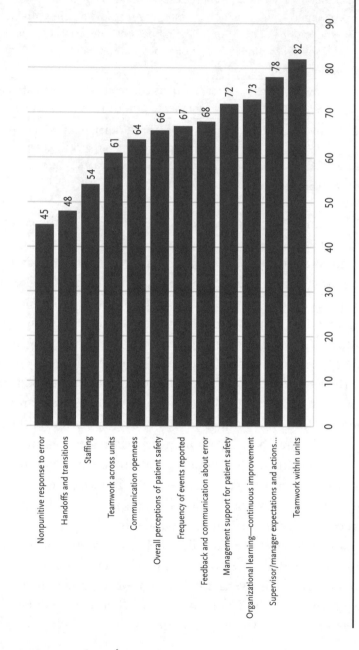

Source: Data from Westat et al. (2016).

KEY TAKEAWAYS

- Leadership is about making employees feel safe and about creating an atmosphere that supports transparency, models acceptance of responsibility, and integrates safety messages into daily activities and meetings without the fear of retribution.
- Good leaders model the way by walking the talk and by giving employees access to the right tools and resources to be successful.
- Dyad leaders at all levels can reduce variation and the propensity for failure by instilling the principles of an HRO and by promoting the values of mutual respect, trust, and teamwork. They support:
  - Open channels of communication based on trust and accountability
  - Proactive prevention of unsafe conditions through education, dashboards, and follow-ups
  - A culture of openness that rejects fear, intimidation, and retribution
  - Infusion of the culture with values of mutual respect, fairness, and learning
  - The use of feedback surveys to gauge attitudes toward safety and develop team training for quality improvement

REFERENCES

Agency for Healthcare Research and Quality (AHRQ). 2019. "Hospital Survey on Patient Safety Culture." Published March. www.ahrq.gov/sops/quality-patient-safety/patientsafetyculture/index.html.

———. 2018. *Hospital Survey on Patient Survey Culture: 2018 Patient Data Report.* US Department of Health and Human

Services. Published March. www.ahrq.gov/sites/default/files/wysiwyg/sops/quality-patient-safety/patientsafetyculture/2018hospitalsopsreport.pdf.

Hines, S., K. Luna, J. Lofthus, M. Marquardt, and D. Stelmokas. 2008. *Becoming a High Reliability Organization: Operational Advice for Hospital Leaders*. Agency for Healthcare Research and Quality. Published April. https://archive.ahrq.gov/professionals/quality-patient-safety/quality-resources/tools/hroadvice/hroadvice.pdf.

James M. Anderson Center for Health Systems Excellence. 2019. "Becoming a High Reliability Organization." Cincinnati Children's. Accessed March 20. www.cincinnatichildrens.org/service/j/anderson-center/safety/methodology/high-reliability.

Joint Commission. 2017. "The Essential Role of Leadership in Developing a Safety Culture." *Sentinel Event Alert*. Published March 1. www.jointcommission.org/assets/1/18/SEA_57_Safety_Culture_Leadership_0317.pdf.

Joint Commission Center for Transforming Healthcare. 2019. "Teaming Up." Accessed March 20. www.centerfortransforminghealthcare.org/teaming_up.aspx.

Westat, R., T. Famolaro, N. Dyer Yount, W. Burns, E. Flashner, H. Liu, and J. Sorra. 2016. *Hospital Survey on Patient Safety Culture: 2016 User Comparative Database Report*. Agency for Healthcare Research and Quality. Published March 2016. www.ahrq.gov/sites/default/files/wysiwyg/professionals/quality-patient-safety/patientsafetyculture/hospital/2016/2016_hospitalsops_report_pt1.pdf.

CHAPTER 17

Teamwork: Assessment and Development

INTRODUCTION

Teamwork plays an important role in the causation and prevention of adverse events. Research has confirmed that staff members' perceptions of teamwork and attitudes toward safety are related directly to safe patient care. The Institute of Medicine (IOM) report *To Err Is Human: Building a Safer Health Care System* indicated that teamwork has a direct effect on patient safety and treatment outcomes (Kohn, Corrigan, and Donaldson 1999).

Teamwork expands the traditional roles of clinicians and staff members to share in the decision-making process. It involves shared responsibility, mutual trust, and enhanced communication. It can take place across units when members cooperate and coordinate with one another to provide the best care for patients. It can also occur within units when staff support each other, treat each other with respect, and work together as a team. When clinical and nonclinical staff collaborate effectively, healthcare teams can improve patient outcomes, prevent medical errors, improve efficiency, and increase patient satisfaction.

TEAMWORK MATTERS FOR ACCOUNTABLE CARE ORGANIZATIONS AND PATIENT-CENTERED MEDICAL HOMES

Accountable care organizations (ACOs) with a strong focus on preventive and postdischarge care, as well as acute care, benefit from collaboration across settings. This type of coordination involves physicians, social workers, nurses with various roles, and case managers as part of multidisciplinary teams. These teams integrate care for targeted populations and communicate medical and social issues to care teams.

Usually, the highest-risk patients involving home health care providers within 48 hours after discharge, readmission, and medication reconciliation are assigned a case manager. Case managers need to coordinate and collaborate across the continuum of care for an ACO model or patient-centered medical homes (PCMHs) to work effectively. The case manager facilitates patients' (and family members') understanding of the care they receive and helps them to stay out of the hospital or emergency department, transitioning back into the community.

A study of medical practices by Ann O'Malley and colleagues (2015) found that a team approach to primary care was fostered by delegating more of physicians' nonclinical tasks to other staff, soliciting staff input on workflow modifications and feeding data back to the team, expanding the roles of medical assistants and nurses, and holding regular team huddles. Delegation engaged staff in workflow redesign and established a safe culture for feedback and questions. In addition, using outside coaches or practice facilitators, huddles, electronic health records (EHR) templates to guide data collection by medical assistants and nurses, and task completion tracking helped prevent sliding back to pre-teamwork behaviors. The study's other key findings included the following:

- Physicians are more willing to delegate when team staffing is stable and delegation is introduced incrementally, starting with routine tasks to medical assistants and licensed practical nurses.
- Assigning roles to team members helps increase their job satisfaction and allows physicians more time to focus on patients' complex needs.
- Facilitation strategies involve huddles for clarifying the day's game plan; colocating the physician, nurse, and medical assistant; promoting a culture in which staff could feel comfortable providing feedback; and taking advantage of EHR functions such as instant messaging and task lists.
- Nurse care managers' roles are central because of their work with patients between physician visits to help manage chronic conditions and develop care plans in partnership with patients and physicians.
- Patients are recognized as partners in identifying health goals, carrying out care plans, self-managing chronic conditions, and making decisions about their care.

The researchers observed that when teams lack formal authority to alter external system challenges (e.g., fee-for-service payment, resources, regulations), they naturally defer to the clinical leadership. Therefore, offering cross-training to potential leaders in how to change care processes may help PCMHs enhance performance and meet patients' needs.

CROSS-TRAINING AND SHARED RESPONSIBILITY

Shared team responsibility implies that all team members work collaboratively toward common goals, review results, and solve problems accountably. Team members, guided by leaders, work interdependently to accomplish common goals.

Cross-training allows members to coach one another or even substitute each other's role. For example, both the nurse and respiratory therapist on a team know how to clear a patient's airway and both share similar levels of competence and confidence in performing this task. They anticipate and support one another's goals and seek each other's unique expertise and perspectives.

Team members are open to feedback about errors and near misses. They listen respectfully to criticism when a member of the team challenges the safety of a plan or a process of care. It means that team members coordinate their work and accept responsibility for outcomes without placing blame.

Dyad leaders are involved in not only coordination and planning, but also in training and development of the team, motivating its members, and supporting a positive atmosphere. Training that follows the IOM core competency of working as an interdisciplinary team also promotes shared understanding and improves interpersonal communication. Training that includes all members of the team has been shown to improve patient outcomes. For example, team training in obstetrics and in gynecology has been shown to prevent errors and improve patient safety (ACOG Committee on Opinion 2009).

PROMOTING TEAMWORK AND OPEN COMMUNICATION

Problems that go undetected or unreported—often because of burnout—are problems that cannot be resolved and could become detrimental. Intimidating behaviors, hostile actions, bullying, and harassment can have a significant negative impact on patients. Reluctance or refusal to answer questions or return calls, condescending language or demeaning comments, or ignoring safety standards stand in stark contrast to the principles of high-reliability organizations. Studies show that clinician burnout is associated with lower perceptions of patient safety culture, and that it can affect patient outcomes directly or indirectly.

Promoting a safety culture cannot occur without a commitment to transparent communications in response to reports of adverse events, near misses, and unsafe conditions. Anticipating the needs of others, adjusting to each other's actions, and adopting a shared understanding of how a procedure is taking place help mitigate risks.

In carrying out a surgical procedure, the roles and responsibilities of the surgeon, anesthesiologist, nurses, surgical assistants, and aides are relatively clear, and adapting to one another's actions and roles occurs fluidly. Coordination of intensive medical services across multiple settings, however, is more complex and could affect patient outcomes as a result of high variability.

TEAMWORK SURVEY

Exhibit 17.1 outlines important behavioral characteristics and definitions of effective teamwork across eight dimensions. These dimensions are reflected in the survey presented in exhibit 17.2. The survey will give you a chance to assess the value that you place on teamwork across the eight dimensions and compare it against what team members think. Another option is to have the team itself evaluate the degree of teamwork they perceive. Typically, this involves asking team members what they currently think about their team in light of the eight dimensions and comparing their responses against where they would like their team. The gap between the responses (current vs. desired) provides important clues about possible training needs, prioritizing and focusing training and education goals in areas that need the most improvement.

Exhibit 17.1: Behavioral Characteristics of Effective Teamwork

Dimension	Mindset	Context	Goal	Focus	Roles	Skills
Team development	Reflection	Group members ask themselves what the purpose of this team is and whether they want to become members. The group leader creates a climate in which people can share ideas and feelings and begin to identify and align with common goals.	Identify team structure and team dynamics	Growth / Resources and capabilities that support the team's interests and goals	Obtain external resources / Shape brand identity, image, and reputation	Persuasion / Effective presentation / Negotiation
Team leadership			Employ situational leadership approaches to managing team performance	Innovation / Flexibility	Identify important trends / Facilitate change	Creative thinking / Intuition / Innovation
Promoting cooperation	Collaboration	The group leader emphasizes the common purpose and establishes norms and standards. The group leader clarifies the process of communication and encourages dialogue and involvement.	Clarify the goals for team members and the roles needed to accomplish these goals	Mentoring / Coaching	Develop members' capacity / Be helpful, considerate, sensitive, approachable, open, and fair	Self-understanding / Active listening / Effective communication / Member development
Facilitation of meetings			Facilitate meetings / Encourage participation in team activities	Engagement / Openness	Build cohesion and teamwork / Manage interpersonal relations	Process orientation / Facilitation of problem-solving communication
Conflict resolution	Analysis	The group leader focuses on interdependence. The leader reduces tensions and conflicts. The leader fosters a sense of ownership and shared team leadership.	Recognize sources of conflict and means to resolve them	Stability / Control	Maintain the structure and flow of information / Be dependable and reliable	Scheduling / Organization / Coordination of efforts / Crisis management
Ethical actions			Distinguish ethical from unethical group decisions and behaviors	Integrity / Quality Improvement	Monitor noncompliant behavior / Evaluate facts and details / Inspect nonconformance	Handling data and forms / Review of and response to routine information
Meeting team goals	Action	Team members are committed to team goals and have a clear understanding of expectations and responsibilities. The group leader provides structures for sharing ideas, synergizing, and initiating action.	Recognize the importance of synergy and integrative solutions	Direction / Goal clarity	Clarify expectations through planning and goal setting / Define roles and tasks / Give instructions	Problem solving / Critical thinking / Communication of vision / Execution
Sustainable excellence		Feedback for improving team performance is used to reward success. Team members are given opportunities to assume leadership.	Support the team goals and the need for joint accountability	Outcome / Evaluation	Be work focused, task oriented, responsible / Rely on motivation and personal drive	Stress management / Time management / Productive labor

Exhibit 17.2: Survey Methodology

Rate how strongly you agree or disagree with each of the following statements by placing your responses twice: one for actual, the other for desired.

1 — *Strongly disagree*
2 — *Disagree*
3 — *Neither agree nor disagree*
4 — *Agree*
5 — *Strongly agree*

		Actual	Desired
Team development	1. I am knowledgeable about the dynamics of team development.		
	2. I help team members establish trusting relationships among themselves as the team evolves and matures.		
	3. I use formal process management procedures (e.g., flow charts) to help the team work more efficiently and productively.		
	AVG		
Team leadership	4. I initiate action to accomplish team goals.		
	5. I have a good sense of the future direction of the team.		
	6. I understand the value of synergy in inspiring team members to develop shared goals.		
	AVG		

(continued)

Exhibit 17.2: Survey Methodology *(continued)*

Promoting cooperation	7. I commit group members to a common goal. 8. I help team members organize around clear roles and shared responsibilities. 9. I promote cooperation through trust and mutual respect.
	AVG
Resolving conflict	10. I suggest alternatives that integrate different viewpoints. 11. I understand the importance of mutual respect and active listening during disagreements. 12. I offer trade-offs to reach agreements over competing ideas or suggestions.
	AVG
Facilitating meetings	13. I develop the agenda and get members' input to clarify priorities. 14. I provide information and handouts. 15. I encourage participation and contributions from all team members.
	AVG
Behaving ethically	16. I place my concern for the group ahead of my concern for myself. 17. I am respectful and sensitive to the other members. 18. I treat members with equal respect regardless of gender differences.
	AVG

(continued)

Exhibit 17.2: Survey Methodology *(continued)*

Sustaining excellence	19. I create opportunities for integrative solutions.
	20. I recognize and reward excellent performance.
	21. I pursue excellence.
	AVG
Meeting goals	22. I know how to use teamwork to derive creative solutions.
	23. I collaborate with others to help improve my communication and listening skills.
	24. I help improve the quality of decision-making.
	AVG

You can conduct the survey at the individual level (having each team member self-assess) to provide insights about perceived personal strengths and weaknesses. At the unit level, members' ratings are aggregated into a single table to assess the perceived strengths and weaknesses of the team as a whole.

The results are typically plotted on a bar chart or spidergram that signifies the differences between actual teamwork profiles and more preferred profiles. Team members or dyad leaders can initiate informed conversations and brainstorm ways to reduce the gap between the two profiles. Examples appear in exhibits 17.3 and 17.4.

Exhibit 17.3 shows the aggregate ratings of team members across the eight composites—or dimensions—of the teamwork survey. The scores are calculated by averaging composite-level percent positive scores across all dimensions. Because the percent positive is displayed as an overall average, scores are weighted equally in their contribution to the calculation of the average. The differences between the current and desired ratings are denoted in percentage for each dimension, helpful for ranking the dimensions. This supports the

Exhibit 17.3: Assessment of Teamwork

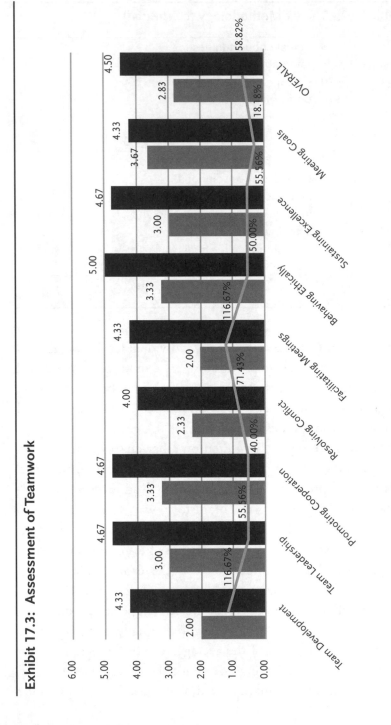

Source: Data from Westat et al. (2016).

Exhibit 17.4: Mapping Teamwork

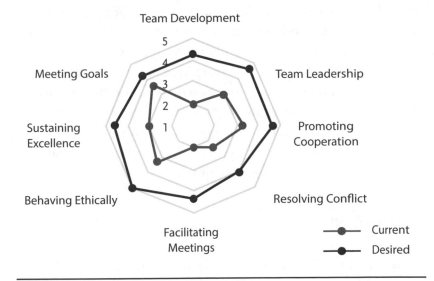

team's effort to develop a meaningful conversation about root causes and brainstorm ideas for further improvement. Dyad leaders, team coordinators, and supervisors can use similar charts to map the responses of members, discuss the results with the team, explore the team's learning experience, and underscore the options for continuous improvement.

Team leadership evolves through transition phases, with each phase characterized by different needs and goals. For example, transitioning from a functional group to a highly interdependent team requires a team charter with goals and objectives, positive attitudes and team norms, clear tasks and metrics, performance strategy, effective communication, trust, and feedback. Moving toward action requires analytics, tracking systems, coordination, engagement, and maintenance of positive relationships and good team performance. To accomplish this, a driving force must be present—a high-impact dyad leadership that is both task oriented and relationship oriented and that has situational skills.

A spidergram in which the gaps between the two sets of ratings are shown holistically appears in exhibit 17.4. It helps to visually detect the differences across the eight dimensions, solicit thoughts and ideas about causes and interventions, prioritize areas for improvement, and agree on a time to review results. For example, both Team Development and Facilitating Meetings reflect much larger "dents" (or gaps) and should be ranked higher on the priority list of team members. Interventions could include team building, goal setting, time management, coaching, and mentoring. Retaking the survey and plotting the results on new diagrams can help the team to review its overall progress over time.

GAINING BUY-IN

Gratton and Erickson (2007) examined 55 large teams that demonstrated high levels of cooperative behaviors despite the complexity of their structures. The researchers isolated eight best practices that correlate with team success. These practices can be applied to transitioning health systems.

1. *Investing in signature relationship practices.* Executives can promote collaborative behavior through personal commitments, championing systemwide efforts, and highly visible statements with supportive communication.
2. *Modeling collaborative behavior.* Teams perform well in organizations where executives switch from silos to systems with interprofessional cooperation and mutual support, regardless of the constraints of disciplinary boundaries.
3. *Creating a gift culture.* Creating incentives for collateral structures of communication and informal networks helps support the social identity of organizational members and encourages them to collaborate.
4. *Ensuring the requisite skills.* Human resources (HR) departments that launch training and education programs

aimed at team building and resolving conflicts have a major impact on the success of teams.

5. *Supporting a strong sense of community.* When executives and HR directors reinforce an adaptive culture that rewards learning and the transfer of best practices across functional lines, organizational members feel more confident in reaching out to others.

6. *Assigning team leaders who are both task-oriented and relationship-oriented.* These roles are complementary and both are important for effective team operations, especially during team transitions through various developmental cycles.

7. *Building on heritage relationships.* Team members who know each other and who develop common understanding and mutual respect over time help promote collaborative behavior.

8. *Understanding role clarity and task ambiguity.* When team members are familiar with the roles and their influence on how the team decides to perform responsibilities or complete tasks, uncertainty and anxiety levels are reduced, adding to the success of the team.

The ability to provide focused care for patients and better population health at a lower cost per capita—with high reliability—requires clinical integration, higher efficiency, effective EHR software and data sharing, and top-notch teamwork.

KEY TAKEAWAYS

- A team approach to primary care is fostered by delegating more of physicians' nonclinical tasks to other staff. Delegation engages staff in workflow redesign and establishes a safe culture for feedback and questions.

- Shared team responsibility implies that all team members collaborate on common goals, review results, and solve problems jointly and accountably.
- Cross-training allows members to coach one another or even substitute for each other's role.
- Dyad leaders are involved in not only coordination and planning but also in team development, guidance, and team motivation.

REFERENCES

ACOG Committee on Opinion. 2009. "Patient Safety in Obstetrics and Gynecology." American College of Obstetricians and Gynecologists. Published December. www.acog.org/Clinical-Guidance-and-Publications/Committee-Opinions/Committee-on-Patient-Safety-and-Quality-Improvement/Patient-Safety-in-Obstetrics-and-Gynecology.

Gratton, L., and T. J. Erickson. 2007. "Eight Ways to Build Collaborative Teams." *Harvard Business Review* 85 (11): 101–9.

Kohn, L. T., J. M. Corrigan, and M. S. Donaldson. 1999. *To Err Is Human: Building a Safer Health System*. Washington, DC: National Academy Press.

O'Malley, A. S., R. Gourevitch, K. Draper, A. Bond, and M. A. Tirodkar. 2015. "Overcoming Challenges to Teamwork in Patient-Centered Medical Homes: A Qualitative Study." *Journal of General Internal Medicine* 30 (2): 183–92.

PART V

Role: Patient Advocate

Exhibit 5: Patient Advocate

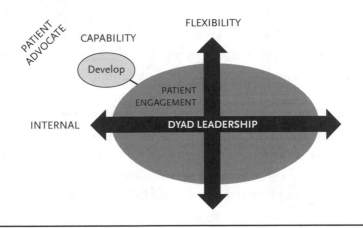

Patient advocacy and doctor–patient communication are crucial for establishing trust between patients and doctors, reducing the number of errors, and ultimately increasing patient satisfaction. From a health policy standpoint, it is imperative that hospital administrators stress open and clear communication between doctors and patients to avoid problems ranging from misdiagnoses to incorrectly followed treatment plans.

Patients who report positive communication with their doctors are likely to communicate pertinent information about their ailments quickly and to adhere to treatment regimens. This leads to an approximately 50 percent reduction in diagnostic tests and referrals, shorter length of stay, fewer complications, strong recovery, and improved emotional health two months after discharge. While investments in training and education for doctors to alter their standard script when communicating with patients is expensive, it is worth the cost—hospital performance ratings and patient satisfaction are likely to increase.

Chapter 18 centers on the critical role of physicians as patient advocates with a primary focus on doctor–patient communication (DPC). The physician is the ultimate patient advocate. Physician advocates may review diagnoses, treatment options, tests, medications, and medical records and assist patients with decision-making. Chapter 19 covers DPC with a focus on communication interaction competencies. Patients want their doctors to be responsive, respectful, confident, empathetic, humane, personal, forthright, and thorough.

Chapter 20 introduces a set of instruments for evaluating the effectiveness of DPC across the eight interaction competencies. Chapter 21 provides a macro view of DPC by examining hospital ratings, an important facet of measuring the patient experience and for determining hospital success and level of reimbursement.

CHAPTER 18

The Context for the Dyad Patient Advocate

INTRODUCTION

Advocating for patients is a core value in patient care. The code of conduct for the American College of Surgeons includes it as a first principle. In informational materials for patients, the Joint Commission reinforced the imperative to clarify the rights of patients and their families to be involved in care (Joint Commission 2019). As a patient, you have the right to

- be informed about the care you will receive;
- get important information about your care in your preferred language;
- get information in a manner that meets your needs, if you have vision, speech, hearing, or mental impairments;
- make decisions about your care;
- refuse care;
- know the names of the caregivers who treat you;
- receive safe care; and
- have your pain addressed.

Patient advocacy is an area of specialization in healthcare. Patient advocates are assigned to patients by hospitals to help them navigate the health system—procedurally, clinically, logistically, and financially.

Well-trained professionals serve as go-betweens for patients and their family members and hospital representatives. They may help people to secure healthcare, manage insurance, make wise financial choices, or make treatment plan decisions. These specialized advocates can locate services to assist patients with independence, find assisted living or nursing home care, or help individuals navigate Medicare while hospitalized or at home. They obtain medical records, ask questions, keep notes, help patients make their own difficult medical decisions, and review and negotiate medical bills.

Advocates can provide guidance with matters such as living wills, advance directives, disability or worker's compensation, or malpractice. Others focus on the care of the elderly.

Options also include the hiring of a nurse, a doctor, or a trained and experienced caregiver by the patient or family members.

TREATING PATIENTS RESPECTFULLY

The physician is the ultimate patient advocate. Physician advocates may review diagnoses, treatment options, tests, medications, and medical records and assist patients with decision-making. In this chapter, we discuss the critical role of physicians as patient advocates with a primary focus on doctor–patient communication (DPC).

A critical factor in the effectiveness of healthcare delivery is sustaining patient centeredness through meaningful DPC. Evidence from research shows that when patient satisfaction is high,

- compliance with medical directives increases,
- predisposition to ask follow-up questions of a provider strengthens,
- the inclination to initiate litigation against a provider decreases, and
- 30-day readmission rates are lower.

Code of Professional Conduct

As Fellows of the American College of Surgeons, we treasure the trust that our patients have placed in us because trust is integral to the practice of surgery. During the continuum of pre-, intra-, and postoperative care, we accept the following responsibilities:

- Serve as effective advocates of our patients' needs
- Disclose therapeutic options, including their risks and benefits
- Disclose and resolve any conflict of interest that might influence decisions regarding care
- Be sensitive and respectful of patients, understanding their vulnerability during the perioperative period
- Fully disclose adverse events and medical errors
- Acknowledge patients' psychological, social, cultural, and spiritual needs
- Encompass within our surgical care the special needs of terminally ill patients
- Acknowledge and support the needs of patients' families
- Respect the knowledge, dignity, and perspective of other healthcare professionals . . .

As surgeons, we acknowledge that we interact with our patients when they are most vulnerable. Their trust and the privileges we enjoy depend on our individual and collective participation in efforts to promote the good of both our patients and society. As Fellows of the American College of Surgeons, we commit ourselves and the College to the ideals of professionalism.

—American College of Surgeons (2016)

Patient advocates may handle complaints about particular treatment plans or healthcare providers that potentially obscure or impede optimal patient care. They facilitate medical encounters, which can be stressful and difficult for individuals (even those in good health) without a medical background, helping patients make the best decision about their healthcare. Some patient advocates may also assist with selecting appropriate insurance, navigating insurance rules, filing and managing insurance claims, and reviewing medical bills. They might offer legal or ethical advocacy.

The benefits of treating patients respectfully are likely to be substantial. Respect engenders trust, and having a trusting relationship allows physicians and patients to work together as partners. Positive outcomes of doctor–patient communication include increased adherence and compliance, adjustment of expectations, self-regulation, and better coping (Matusitz and Spear 2014). Effective communication with patients has the potential to help mitigate anxiety; control emotions; facilitate meaningful exchange of medical information; and allow for a better understanding of patients' needs, perceptions, and expectations.

Meaningful DPC can enhance patient satisfaction and adherence and contribute to patients' understanding of their illnesses and the risks and benefits of treatment. What's more, optimizing communication can lead to better patient health and outcomes for patients and hospitals and even to reduced malpractice suits. Researchers have noted that many malpractice suits are brought not because of complaints about the quality of medical care but as an expression of anger about some aspects of doctor–patient communications (Bernard et al. 1999). Physicians who understand and who respond appropriately to the emotional needs of their patients are less likely to be sued. Thus, efforts to improve physicians' training should include empathy and interpersonal communication skills (Hammerly, Harmon, and Schwaitzberg 2014). This chapter addresses skill development in subsequent sections.

FALLING THROUGH THE CRACKS

Communication with medical staff and clinicians, however, can be daunting, if not impossible—especially during transitions, when shift changes may involve interactions with different doctors and nurses. Gaps in communication may occur because of uneasiness or limited time or interest. Communication skills tend to decline as medical students progress through their medical education and, over time, doctors (especially in highly specialized fields) tend to lose their focus on holistic patient care.

Physicians often tend to overestimate their ability to communicate in interpersonal exchanges by considering the communication adequate or even effective while patients feel otherwise. Tongue, Epps, and Forese (2005) reported that 75 percent of the orthopedic surgeons surveyed in their sample believed that they communicated satisfactorily with their patients, but only 21 percent of the patients reported satisfactory communication with their doctors.

Primary care physicians, especially under the pressures of time constraints, overscheduling, and patients' wait-time complaints, often use less-than-thorough communications, leaving patients at risk of mistreatments or preventable readmissions. In a study of primary care physicians and surgeons, Braddock and colleagues (1999) reviewed audiotapes of informed decision-making and found that discussion of alternatives occurred in 5.5– 29.5 percent of interactions, of pros and cons in 2.3–6.3 percent, and of uncertainties associated with the decision in 1.1–16.6 percent. However, physicians rarely explored whether patients understood their decision (0.9–6.9 percent).

Every so often, physicians deflect patients' concerns and expectations for more information. Alexander, Casalino, and Metzler (2003) found that while 63 percent of the patients have expressed a need to talk with their physicians about out-of-pocket costs, and 79 percent of the physicians felt these conversations were important, only 35 percent of physicians and 15 percent of patients reported having these conversations.

Patients and physicians often cite discomfort, insufficient time, patients' belief that their physicians do not have a viable solution, and concerns about the impact of the conversations on quality of care. Thus, despite the mutual understanding that physician–patient communication about healthcare costs is important, little such communication occurs.

NONADHERENCE

Ineffective DPC is problematic as it can lead to nonadherence and other health-related issues such as the stress of paying for medical expenses. Medication nonadherence is an important public health consideration, affecting health outcomes and overall healthcare costs. In the United States, about 50 percent of the 3.2 billion annual prescriptions dispended for chronic disease are not taken as prescribed. The Agency for Health Research and Quality attributes low medication adherence rates to the following factors:

- Poor communication between the provider and patient or family
- Socioeconomic barriers for the patient
- Complexity of medication regimen prescribed (Williams 2014)

If left unchecked, the high prevalence of medication nonadherence may have a substantial and detrimental impact on US population health and economic progress. Nonadherence causes approximately 125,000 deaths and at least 10 percent of hospitalizations; it costs the already-strained healthcare system anywhere from $100 billion to $289 billion a year (Boylan 2017).

FORMAL EDUCATION

Some schools of medicine provide training to medical students to become better patient advocates. The Advocacy Training Program at the Boston University Medical Campus, for example, trains medical students to advocate for the health and well-being of patients and their communities (Hopkins 2013). About 15 percent of students in each class participate. Some of them go on to teach in the program, mastering content and resources and acquiring the skills and techniques necessary to teach. They also become mentors to fellow students.

The program comprises a first-year course focused on the social determinants of health (taught by students who have taken the course and faculty engaged in advocacy) and a second-year course with a focus on interdisciplinary learning, taught by students in medicine and law and by and physicians and lawyers engaged in advocacy. In the third year, students learn from case-based online modules related to the rotations they are taking that year; in the fourth year, they choose an advocacy project and carry it out with the mentorship of a faculty member.

KEY TAKEAWAYS

- Medication nonadherence poses a threat to public health and increases costs of healthcare.
- Many malpractice suits are brought not because of complaints about the quality of medical care but as an expression of frustration about some aspects of DPC.
- A critical factor in the effectiveness of healthcare delivery is sustaining patient centeredness.
- Meaningful DPC can enhance patient satisfaction and adherence.

- Respect, empathy, and the opportunity to give feedback contribute to patients' understanding of illness and the risks and benefits of treatment, lowering the probability of malpractice suits.

REFERENCES

Alexander, G. C., L. P. Casalino, and D. O. Meltzer. 2003. "Patient–Physician Communication About Out-of-Pocket Costs." *Journal of the American Medical Association* 290 (7): 953–58.

American College of Surgeons. 2016. "Code of Professional Conduct." Revised April 12. www.facs.org/about-acs/statements/stonprin#code.

Bernard, B., B. Virshup, A. Oppenberg, and M. Coleman. 1999. "Strategic Risk Management: Reducing Malpractice Claims Through More Effective Patient–Doctor Communication." *American Journal of Medical Quality* 14 (4): 153–59.

Boylan, L. 2017. "The Cost of Medication Non-adherence." National Association of Chain Drug Stores. Published April 20. www.nacds.org/news/the-cost-of-medication-non-adherence.

Braddock, C. H., K. A. Edwards, N. M. Hasenberg, T. L. Laidley, and W. Levinson. 1999. "Informed Decision Making in Outpatient Practice: Time to Get Back to Basics." *Journal of the American Medical Association* 282 (24): 2313–20.

Hammerly, M. E., L. Harmon, and S. D. Schwaitzberg. 2014. "Good to Great: Using 360-Degree Feedback to Improve Physician Emotional Intelligence." *Journal of Healthcare Management* 59 (5): 354–65.

Hopkins, M. 2013. "Training MED Students to Become Patient Advocates." *BU Today*. Published January 14. www.bu.edu/today/2013/training-med-students-to-become-patient-advocates/.

Joint Commission. 2019. "Speak Up." Accessed March 21. www.jointcommission.org/assets/1/6/Know_Your_Rights_brochure.pdf.

Matusitz, J., and J. Spear. 2014. "Effective Doctor–Patient Communication: An Updated Examination." *Social Work in Public Health* 29 (3): 252–66.

Tongue, J. R., H. R. Epps, and L. L. Forese. 2005. "Communication Skills for Patient-Centered Care: Research-Based, Easily Learned Techniques for Medical Interviews That Benefit Orthopedic Surgeons and Their Patients." *Journal of Bone and Joint Surgery* 87 (3): 652–58.

Williams, A. 2014. "Issue Brief: Medication Adherence and Health IT." Office of the National Coordinator for Health Information Technology. Published January 9. www.healthit.gov/sites/default/files/medicationadherence_and_hit_issue_brief.pdf.

CHAPTER 19

Doctor–Patient Communication

INTRODUCTION

A physician's interpersonal communication skills encompass the ability to gather information to facilitate accurate diagnoses, counsel appropriately, provide therapeutic instructions, and establish trusting relationships. To create trust and increase medication adherence, doctors should give feedback while establishing a warm atmosphere, acceptance, and empathy.

This chapter introduces a tool for assessing physicians' communication competence. The DPCA, or Doctor–Patient Communication Assessment, is consistent with the frameworks developed in this book. The objective of the DPCA is also consistent with the need to maintain a shared understanding of patients' health conditions for effective validation and therapeutic rapport (Mira et al. 2014; Norfolk, Birdi, and Patterson 2009).

BLIND SPOTS, SWEET SPOTS

The DPCA is aimed at gauging the effectiveness of the interpersonal communication and capturing patients' perceptions of the quality of care and service they receive.

The assessment is used at the individual or group level, typically as part of a formal training program that also includes intervention and development. At the individual level, the assessment can be conducted by physicians to examine how they perceive their interactions with patients (Actual) as compared to how well they would like to carry out these interactions (Ideal). Alternatively, the surveys can be adapted to allow patients to evaluate their interpersonal communication with their care providers. The gap between the two results informs physicians and hospital leaders about possible glitches or discrepancies between blind spots and sweet spots.

Patients want their physicians to be responsive, respectful, confident, empathetic, humane, personal, forthright, and thorough. Subtle gestures, body language, eye contact, paraverbal cues, and nonverbal cues are judged critically by patients. These elements of conversation form their perceptions about the overall value of their medical encounter.

Blind spots, or the behavioral and perceptual areas known to patients but unknown to physicians, provide clues about how to maintain a good balance and avoid poor communication or forms of behavior considered to be dysfunctional. Sweet spots represent good balance or alignment between the perceived responses. While physicians receive personal feedback from the tool about their interactions, including an understanding that highlights areas for self-improvement, the hospital receives aggregate feedback (i.e., surveys of all doctor–patient communications, or DPCs) that shows the overall trajectory of improvement over time.

COMPETENCIES

The DPCA is based on an interpersonal communication framework that highlights eight competencies and sensitivity skills essential for effective provider–patient interactions. Together they cover verbal and nonverbal communication, effective questioning and transmission of information (task-oriented behavior), expressions of empathy and concerns (psychosocial behavior), consultation, and joint decision-making. The eight competencies include the following:

1. *Respecting.* Greeting patients warmly and acknowledging that patients deserve prompt answers so they can make decisions regarding their care.
2. *Interacting.* Conveying meaning nonverbally through subtle cues that complement and illustrate aspects of the verbal interaction.
3. *Empathizing.* Expressing emotional understanding or feelings about patients' concerns and engaging or empowering patients to take charge of their health.
4. *Listening.* Asking the right questions and actively listening to patients by showing respect for their self-knowledge and building trust.
5. *Validating.* Recognizing and accepting patients' thoughts, feelings, sensations, and behaviors.
6. *Sense making.* Diagnosing and treating patients, anticipating complications, recognizing changes in patients' reactions, and communicating effectively during care transitions.
7. *Facilitating.* Interacting meaningfully with patients to minimize anxiety associated with considerable stress.
8. *Counseling.* Enhancing communication and education to improve patient knowledge, adherence, and correct use of medication.

DIMENSIONS

These eight competencies are grouped into four dimensions, or composites, that signify the boundaries for physician–patient communication:

1. *Nonverbal communication.* This includes gestures, facial expressions, body movement, timing, touch, and anything else done without speaking. *Paraverbal* communication involves messages transmitted through the tone, pitch, and pacing of our voices (e.g., happy, sad, angry, determined, forceful).
2. *Empathy.* This is the emotional understanding of others' feelings and concerns.
3. *Attentiveness.* This consists of responsiveness to patients' concerns and issues.
4. *Consultation.* This is essential for examining and identifying options through common understanding and acceptance.

Tone of voice and the way by which individuals choose words are important considerations in DPC. Anecdotally, 55 percent of communication is transmitted via body language, 38 percent involves the tone of voice, and 7 percent reflects the actual words spoken (Thompson 2011). Some formal studies have found that 90 percent of the meaning in interpersonal communication derives from non-verbal signals, and more recent and reliable findings claim that it is closer to 65 percent (Guerrero and Floyd 2006).

Patients may rely more on nonverbal cues in medical encounters when verbal and nonverbal messages are inconsistent and during direct consultation when emotional or relational communication is taking place (Hargie 2011). For example, when a patient asks a question and the care provider is nonspecific about the approach or direction, patients may look for nonverbal cues to fill in the void.

METHODOLOGY AND DATA COLLECTION FOR ASSESSING DOCTOR–PATIENT COMMUNICATION

The 32 questions in exhibit 19.1 are distributed across the 4 categories (nonverbal communication, empathy, attentiveness, consultation) and 8 competencies. Together, they reflect the communication relationship between doctors and patients. The self-assessment elicits physicians' (actual and ideal) responses to the survey questions.

ANALYSIS AND INTERPRETATION

Scores between 5 and 6 indicate an appreciation of the underlying values in each quadrant. The scores also show a greater ability to recognize and employ effective communication skills and the ability to integrate the behaviors and use the competencies in complementary ways.

Scores between 2 and 3 indicate areas of weakness and the potential for skill building. Scores approaching four imply that the physician is comfortable in some areas and uncomfortable in others. Note how the chart displaying *actual* behaviors in exhibit 19.2 "caves in" in some areas. In general, these gaps are targeted for self-improvement.

QUADRANTS

The next cluster of assessments depicts the quadrants, or four dimensions, in which the exchange of communication between doctors and patients occur. Doctors provide verbal and nonverbal assurances to patients and establish the trust necessary for treatment adherence.

Developing sensitivity to ethnicity in intercultural physician–patient interactions and building trust are of utmost importance. Cultural competence—the ability of providers and organizations to effectively deliver healthcare services that meet the social, cultural, and linguistic needs of patients—is essential for removing potential barriers to effective communication. Nonverbal and paraverbal responses by physicians are illustrated in exhibit 19.3. The expression of the physicians' emotional understanding of patients' feelings appears in exhibit 19.4. Physicians' responses to patients' concerns and issues are illustrated in exhibit 19.5. Finally, exhibit 19.6 shows

Exhibit 19.1: Survey Methodology for Doctor–Patient Communication Assessment

Frequency Level (Seven-Point Likert Scale)
Next to each statement indicate the response that best matches your situation.

1 — *Never*
2 — *Rarely (in fewer than 10 percent of my chances)*
3 — *Occasionally (in about 30 percent of my chances)*
4 — *Sometimes (in about 50 percent of my chances)*
5 — *Frequently (in about 70 percent of my chances)*
6 — *Usually (in about 90 percent of my chances)*
7 — *Every time*

Quadrants	Competencies	Behavioral Indicators	Actual	Ideal
		1. I greet my patients warmly by name.		
		2. I respect the confidentiality of patients.		
	Respecting	3. I provide a useful space and time to talk with patients about their care.		
		4. I answer every question thoroughly and respectfully.		
		AVG		
Nonverbal communication		5. I establish eye contact with the patient when entering the room.		
		6. I greet patients with a warm and welcoming smile.		
	Interacting	7. I use welcoming body language to gain trust.		
		8. I use nonverbal communication to convey a sense of warmth, empathy, caring, reassurance, and support.		
		AVG		

(continued)

Exhibit 19.1: Survey Methodology for Doctor–Patient Communication Assessment *(continued)*

Empathy	Empathizing	9. I create a comforting environment to reduce stress.
		10. I calm patients' fears and concerns.
		11. I show patients that I am familiar with their past medical history.
		12. I allow the time needed for patients to comprehend the new information.
		AVG
	Listening	13. I carefully listen to patients' questions and concerns.
		14. I encourage patients to talk about their concerns.
		15. I ask patients about the benefits or side effects of previous medication.
		16. I solicit more questions before leaving the exam room.
		AVG
Attentiveness	Validating	17. I regularly inquire whether my patients understand what I say or do during the exam.
		18. I encourage questions to help patients understand their own healthcare issues.
		19. I ask patients for specific feedback about medication adherence.
		20. After discharge, I make sure patients understand and follow home care instructions.
		AVG

(continued)

Attentiveness	Sense making	21. I assess the symptoms experienced and their impact on patients' lives.
		22. I routinely ask patients about previous reactions to medications or tests.
		23. I ask patients for specific feedback about medication adherence.
		24. I encourage patients to ask additional questions.
		AVG
Consultation	Facilitating	25. I review the patient's chart before entering the examination room.
		26. I make sure patients are aware that I know about the long wait time.
		27. I allocate sufficient time for patient participation.
		28. I make sure patients know how to reach me or another doctor if they have questions after discharge.
		AVG
	Counseling	29. I clarify the risks, benefits, and compliance issues of choosing a treatment.
		30. I discuss all possible adverse effects.
		31. I communicate the side effects of a new medication.
		32. I give patients the information to make informed decisions about treatment and care.
		AVG

Exhibit 19.2: Doctor–Patient Communication Assessment

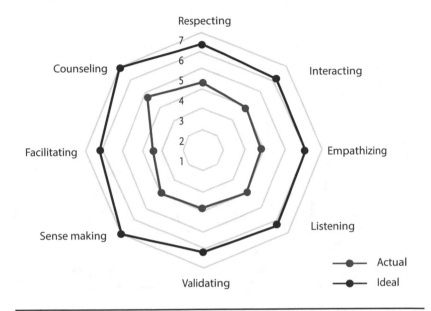

the sensitivity of physicians to the need to include patients in consultation and joint decision-making.

Physicians tend to rely on a scripted communication style using uninterrupted narratives, which gives patients limited opportunity to ask questions until the end. This style reduces their ability to adapt messages culturally or individually—it is not as effective as shared interviews to affect behavioral change (Matusitz and Spear 2014).

By recognizing and addressing the gaps revealed by the survey, physicians can develop better relationships with patients—for example, paying close attention to personal attitudes and their effects on patients' perceptions of fairness, equity, and privacy. Moreover, though researchers have found that patients prefer the physician to

Exhibit 19.3: Nonverbal

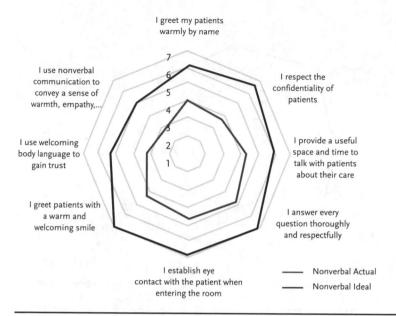

I greet my patients warmly by name

I use nonverbal communication to convey a sense of warmth, empathy,...

I respect the confidentiality of patients

I use welcoming body language to gain trust

I provide a useful space and time to talk with patients about their care

I greet patients with a warm and welcoming smile

I answer every question thoroughly and respectfully

I establish eye contact with the patient when entering the room

—— Nonverbal Actual
—— Nonverbal Ideal

Exhibit 19.4: Empathy

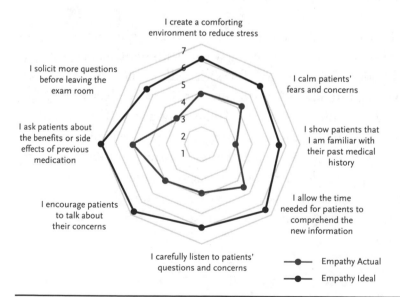

I create a comforting environment to reduce stress

I solicit more questions before leaving the exam room

I calm patients' fears and concerns

I ask patients about the benefits or side effects of previous medication

I show patients that I am familiar with their past medical history

I encourage patients to talk about their concerns

I allow the time needed for patients to comprehend the new information

I carefully listen to patients' questions and concerns

—●— Empathy Actual
—●— Empathy Ideal

Exhibit 19.5: Attentiveness

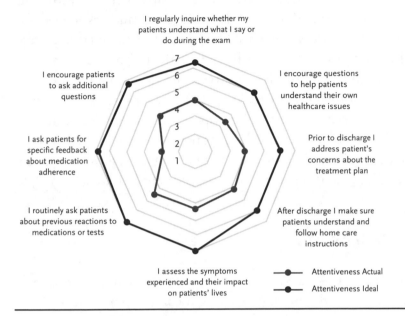

I regularly inquire whether my patients understand what I say or do during the exam

I encourage patients to ask additional questions

I encourage questions to help patients understand their own healthcare issues

I ask patients for specific feedback about medication adherence

Prior to discharge I address patient's concerns about the treatment plan

I routinely ask patients about previous reactions to medications or tests

After discharge I make sure patients understand and follow home care instructions

I assess the symptoms experienced and their impact on patients' lives

—●— Attentiveness Actual
—●— Attentiveness Ideal

Exhibit 19.6: Consultation

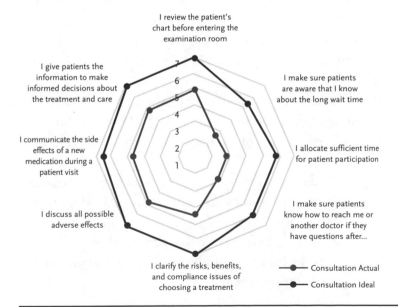

I review the patient's chart before entering the examination room

I give patients the information to make informed decisions about the treatment and care

I make sure patients are aware that I know about the long wait time

I communicate the side effects of a new medication during a patient visit

I allocate sufficient time for patient participation

I discuss all possible adverse effects

I make sure patients know how to reach me or another doctor if they have questions after...

I clarify the risks, benefits, and compliance issues of choosing a treatment

—●— Consultation Actual
—●— Consultation Ideal

be in charge (Street and Millay 2001), care providers have an opportunity to improve their interpersonal competencies by providing confirming information, exhibiting sensitivity, and acknowledging or alleviating patient concerns. Physicians can encourage openness, invite questions, and actively listen to patients. They can rely more on interactive communication styles and develop a broader perspective that includes the sociopsychological and physical needs of patients, enabling honest and transparent doctor–patient consultation. Empowering and involving patients actively in the decision-making process establishes an environment of trust, promotes patient centeredness, and ultimately increases patient satisfaction.

KEY TAKEAWAYS

- The DPCA is based on an interpersonal communication framework that highlights eight competencies and sensitivity skills essential for effective provider–patient interactions.
- The DPCA covers verbal and nonverbal communication, effective questioning and transmission of information (task-oriented behavior), expressions of empathy and concerns (psychosocial behavior), consultation, and joint decision-making.
- The assessment is aimed at gauging the effectiveness of the interpersonal communication, as well as at capturing patients' perceptions of the quality of the care and services they receive.
- Gaps provide clues about how to maintain a good balance and avoid poor communication or perceived dysfunctional forms of behavior.
- Physicians receive personal feedback about their interactions, including an understanding that highlights areas for self-improvement.

- Hospitals receive aggregate feedback (i.e., ratings from all DPC surveys) that shows the overall trajectory of improvement of DPC ratings over time.

REFERENCES

Guerrero, L. K., and K. Floyd. 2006. *Nonverbal Communication in Close Relationships*. Mahwah, NJ: Lawrence Erlbaum Associates.

Hargie, O. 2011. *Skilled Interpersonal Communication: Research, Theory and Practice*. London, UK: Routledge.

Matusitz, J., and J. Spear. 2014. "Effective Doctor–Patient Communication: An Updated Examination." *Social Work in Public Health* 29 (3): 252–66.

Mira, J. J., M. Guilabert, V. Pérez-Jover, and S. Lorenzo. 2014. "Barriers for an Effective Communication Around Clinical Decision Making: An Analysis of the Gaps Between Doctors' and Patients' Point of View." *Health Expectations* 17 (6): 826–39.

Norfolk, T., K. Birdi, and F. Patterson. 2009. "Developing Therapeutic Rapport: A Training Validation Study." *Quality in Primary Care* 17 (2): 99–106.

Street, R. L., and B. Millay. 2001. "Analyzing Patient Participation in Medical Encounters." *Health Communication* 13 (1): 61–73.

Thompson, J. 2011. "Is Nonverbal Communication a Numbers Game?" *Psychology Today*. Published September 30. www.psychologytoday.com/blog/beyond-words/201109/is-nonverbal-communication-numbers-game.

CHAPTER 20

Interaction Competencies

INTRODUCTION

All too often physicians tend to overestimate their ability to communicate. They sometimes consider their conversations with patients to be adequate even when the patients themselves are dissatisfied. Increasingly, however, the evidence has shown that physician–patient communication and patient satisfaction are strongly related to quality of care (Manary et al. 2013). The instruments discussed in this chapter provide detail on physician–patient communication by assessing interaction competencies.

ASSESSMENT OF INTERACTION COMPETENCIES

Exhibits 20.1–20.8 reflect potential gaps between the perceived current level of competencies and the desired levels. The scores reflect the behavioral responses of physicians to the items that are included in exhibit 19.1. The differences between these charts reflect opportunities for self-improvement.

A physician's communication and interpersonal skills should go beyond the doctor–patient relationship to encompass the goals of treatment, shared perceptions and feelings regarding the nature of the problem, and sociopsychological support. Patient-centric care is a clinical treatment provided by medical professionals that focuses on respecting and attending to patient preferences, desires, and values.

Exhibit 20.1: Respecting

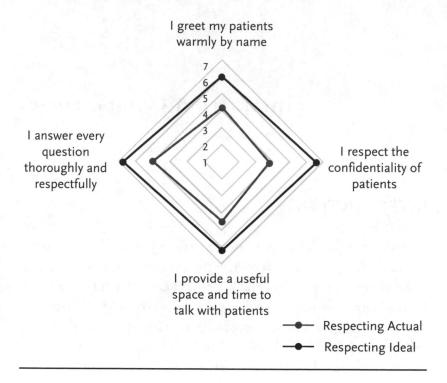

Exhibit 20.2: Interacting

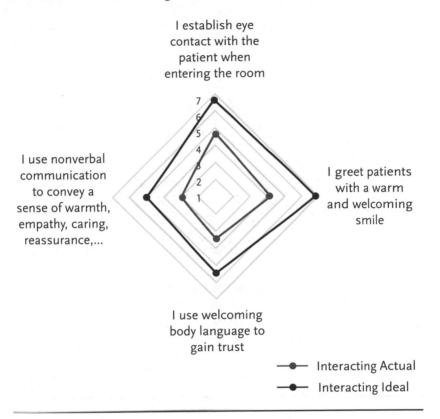

I establish eye contact with the patient when entering the room

I use nonverbal communication to convey a sense of warmth, empathy, caring, reassurance,...

I greet patients with a warm and welcoming smile

I use welcoming body language to gain trust

Interacting Actual
Interacting Ideal

Exhibit 20.3: Empathizing

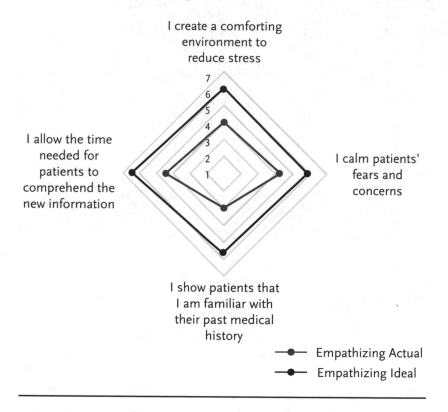

I create a comforting
environment to
reduce stress

I allow the time
needed for
patients to
comprehend the
new information

I calm patients'
fears and
concerns

I show patients that
I am familiar with
their past medical
history

● Empathizing Actual
● Empathizing Ideal

Exhibit 20.4: Listening

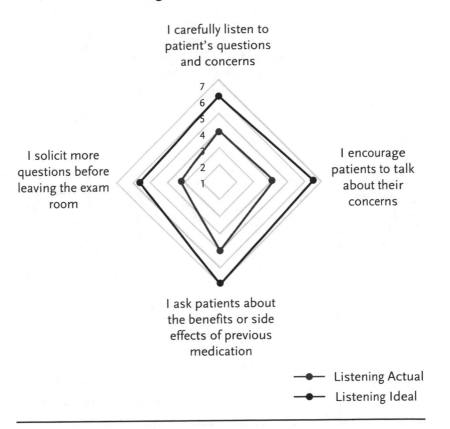

I carefully listen to
patient's questions
and concerns

7
6
5
4
3
2
1

I solicit more
questions before
leaving the exam
room

I encourage
patients to talk
about their
concerns

I ask patients about
the benefits or side
effects of previous
medication

——●—— Listening Actual
——●—— Listening Ideal

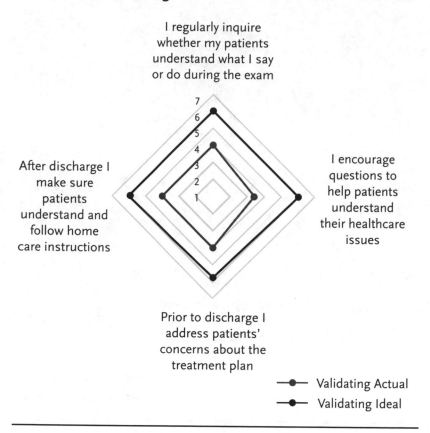

I regularly inquire
whether my patients
understand what I say
or do during the exam

After discharge I
make sure
patients
understand and
follow home
care instructions

I encourage
questions to
help patients
understand
their healthcare
issues

Prior to discharge I
address patients'
concerns about the
treatment plan

—●— Validating Actual
—●— Validating Ideal

Exhibit 20.6: Sense Making

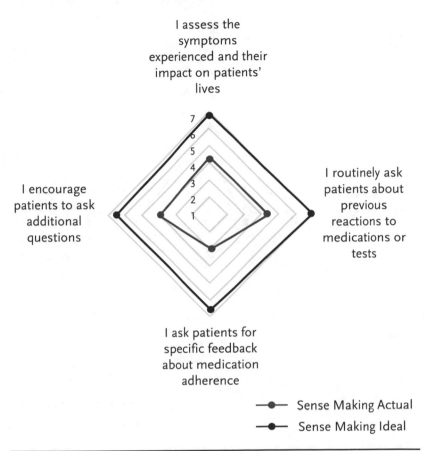

I assess the
symptoms
experienced and their
impact on patients'
lives

I routinely ask
patients about
previous
reactions to
medications or
tests

I encourage
patients to ask
additional
questions

I ask patients for
specific feedback
about medication
adherence

●——— Sense Making Actual
●——— Sense Making Ideal

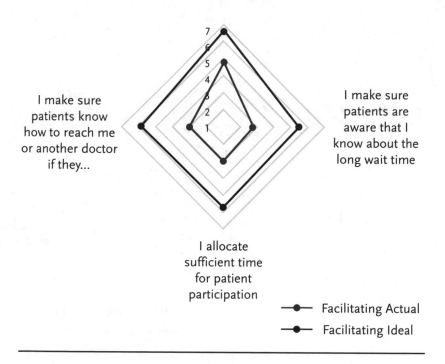

I review the
patient's chart
before entering
the examination...

I make sure
patients know
how to reach me
or another doctor
if they...

I make sure
patients are
aware that I
know about the
long wait time

I allocate
sufficient time
for patient
participation

——●—— Facilitating Actual
——●—— Facilitating Ideal

Exhibit 20.8: Counseling

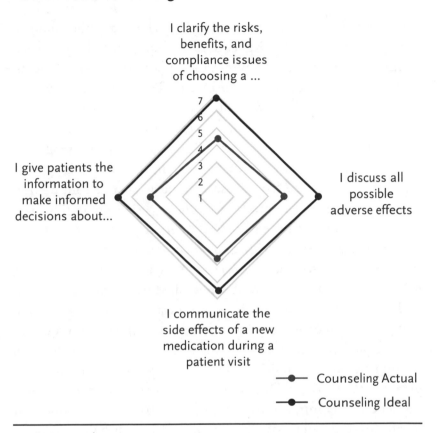

I clarify the risks, benefits, and compliance issues of choosing a ...

I give patients the information to make informed decisions about...

I discuss all possible adverse effects

I communicate the side effects of a new medication during a patient visit

7
6
5
4
3
2
1

Counseling Actual
Counseling Ideal

COMMUNICATION TRAINING

Patient centeredness is sustained through the ability to gather information to facilitate accurate diagnoses, counsel appropriately, give therapeutic instructions, and establish caring relationships with patients.

When a sufficient amount of Doctor–Patient Communication Assessment (DPCA) training is initiated, a norming procedure could be developed and a database may be employed to demonstrate the efficacy of the training program—a critical factor in establishing the credibility of the measurement program and nurturing support for its use. The DPCA could also become a valuable communication training and self-improvement tool, as patients reporting good communication with their doctors are more likely to be satisfied with their care. When satisfied, patients are especially prepared to share pertinent information for accurate diagnosis of their problems, follow advice, and adhere to the prescribed treatment.

In fact, a meta-analysis of 127 studies supports the proposition that patient adherence significantly relates to the communication training of physicians and that adherence and self-management can be improved when physicians are well trained to be better communicators (Haskard and DiMatteo 2009). Other studies have shown that effective communication triggers the patient's commitment to quality care, adherence, follow-ups, and an overall increase in patient satisfaction (Verlinde et al. 2012). This may require a cultural transformation in hospitals—and even community health systems and multispecialty groups—because hospitals have traditionally been slow to adapt to change. Transformation has particularly proven a problem within disciplines that are less collegial or cohesive and with lower organizational identity and trust (Curoe, Kralewski, and Kaissi 2003).

SOFT SKILLS AND CLOSED-LOOP COMMUNICATION

Soft skills include a wide range of interpersonal and social skills and competencies transferable across disciplines and organizational lines. These soft skills include communication, teamwork, problem solving, critical thinking, innovation and creativity, self-confidence, ethical understanding, accepting personal accountability, lifelong learning, and dealing with uncertainty. Dyad leaders, in the role of patient advocates, hone these skills to better adapt to the hospital culture, initiate change and innovation, and contribute to patient care.

Effective teams prevent communication problems by using closed-loop communication, a variant of active listening. Closed-loop communication has been shown to reduce error rates by removing ambiguity and allowing questions if the instructions are not clear. Each verbal communication is addressed to a designated person, who in turn repeats the message back to the sender. This is a requirement to prevent errors from occurring—there is no confusion about what is needed or who is assigned to perform the task. A surgeon gives verbal instruction: "Amanda, hang another unit of blood." Amanda replies, "Hanging another unit of blood" while performing the task. Amanda has restated the message to confirm that she heard and understood it and is doing what is asked. Once she completed the task, she states to the group that the task was completed.

Mutual trust and accountability are key components of the shared approach. Each team member knows from experience that other members will perform their tasks, share information, admit mistakes, and work together to eliminate medical errors. Members are willing to accept constructive intervention to stop anyone from making a mistake, regardless of that person's role on the team.

KEY TAKEAWAYS

- Evidence has shown that doctor–patient communication and patient satisfaction are both significantly related to quality of care.
- Patient-centric care is a clinical treatment provided by medical professionals that focuses on respecting and attending to patient preferences, desires, and values.
- When a sufficient amount of DPCA training is provided, a norming procedure could be developed, and a database may be employed to demonstrate the efficacy of the training program, a critical factor in establishing the credibility of the measurement program and nurturing support for its use.
- In addition to applied learning and functional skills, dyad leaders acting in the role of patient advocates should have a shared capacity that includes
  - entrepreneurial skills to identify creative solutions to problems,
  - clear communication,
  - behavioral flexibility,
  - understanding and resolving conflict, and
  - collaborating with others.

REFERENCES

Curoe, A., J. Kralewski, and A. Kaissi. 2003. "Assessing the Cultures of Medical Group Practices." *Journal of the American Board of Family Medicine* 16 (5): 394–98.

Haskard, Z., and R. M. DiMatteo. 2009. "Physician Communication and Patient Adherence to Treatment: A Meta-analysis." *Medical Care* 47 (8): 826–34.

Manary, M. P., W. Boulding, R. Staelin, and S. W. Glickman. 2013. "The Patient Experience and Health Outcomes." *New England Journal of Medicine* 368 (3): 201–3.

Verlinde, E., N. De Laender, S. De Maesschalck, M. Deveugele, and S. Willems. 2012. "The Social Gradient in Doctor–Patient Communication." *Equity Health Journal* 11: 12.

CHAPTER 21

Hospital Consumer Assessment of Healthcare Providers and Systems

INTRODUCTION

The goal of the Hospital Consumer Assessment of Healthcare Providers and Systems (HCAHPS) is to promote consumer choice, public accountability, and greater transparency in healthcare. The HCAHPS survey contains 21 patient perspectives on care and patient rating items that encompass the 11 composite measures.

Hospitals and healthcare systems are required to survey their admitted patients throughout each month of the year properly and consistently, with a goal of at least 300 completed surveys for each hospital per year, to achieve high reliability for the reported measures. Daily, more than 30,000 patients receive the HCAHPS survey about their recent hospital experience, and more than 8,400 patients complete it (Agency for Healthcare Research and Quality 2017). Eligible patients are those who are 18 years or older on admission; have a non-psychiatric primary discharge diagnosis for medical, surgical, or maternity care; have an overnight stay (or longer) at the hospital under inpatient status (as opposed to observation status); and are alive at discharge. Patients discharged to hospice, prisoners, and patients with foreign home addresses are excluded.

Hospitals may administer the survey themselves or use an approved survey vendor. Hospitals can choose the method for administering the survey—mail only, telephone only, mail with telephone follow-up, or interactive voice-response phone calls. Eligible patients are contacted between 48 hours and six weeks after discharge, and they have six weeks following the initial contact to complete the survey.

KEY PERCENTILES

Exhibit 21.1 displays the key percentiles for each of the 11 publicly reported HCAHPS measures. Both "top box" (most positive) and "bottom box" (least positive) values are shown at the 5th, 10th, 25th, 50th, 75th, 90th, and 95th percentiles.

Using the HCAHPS percentiles table (Health Services Advisory Group 2019), hospital decision makers can easily see where their hospital ranks relative to other hospitals on each of the following HCAHPS measures:

1. Communication with doctors
2. Communication with nurses
3. Responsiveness of hospital staff
4. Pain management
5. Communication about medicines
6. Discharge information
7. Care transition
8. Cleanliness of the hospital environment
9. Quietness of the hospital environment
10. Hospital rating
11. Recommended the hospital

IMPACT OF DOCTOR–PATIENT COMMUNICATION ON HOSPITAL RATINGS

Doctor–patient communication (DPC) is important not only for its impact on patient outcomes but also because of its role in influencing the overall patient ratings of the hospital. Research by Clever and

Exhibit 21.1: HCHAPS Percentiles, December 2017

Hospital Percentile*	Communication with Nurses	Communication with Doctors	Responsiveness of Hosp. Staff	Pain Management	Comm. About Medicines	Cleanliness of Hospital Env.	Quietness of Hospital Env.	Discharge Information	Care Transition	Hospital Rating	Recommend the Hospital
					TOP-Box Score[1]						
95th (near best)	90	92	86	82	79	89	81	93	65	87	88
90th	87	89	82	79	75	85	76	92	61	84	84
75th	84	85	74	74	69	80	69	90	56	78	79
50th	80	82	67	71	64	74	62	88	52	73	73
25th	77	78	62	68	61	69	55	85	48	67	66
10th	74	76	58	64	58	64	49	82	44	62	60
5th (near worst)	72	74	55	62	55	62	46	80	41	58	56
					BOTTOM-Box Score[2]						
5th (near best)	1	0	1	1	7	1	1	7	2	2	0
10th	1	1	3	3	10	3	3	8	2	3	1
25th	2	3	5	5	14	5	5	10	4	5	3
50th	4	4	8	6	18	8	8	12	5	7	4
75th	5	5	11	8	20	11	12	15	6	9	6
90th	7	7	14	10	24	14	16	18	8	12	9
95th (near worst)	9	8	17	12	26	16	19	20	9	14	11

*These results encompass all hospitals that received HCAHPS scores. Because not all hospitals report their results on Hospital Compare, the values on that Web site may differ from those shown here.

*Percentiles for HCAHPS "Top-box" and "Bottom-box" scores of the 4,219 hospitals publicly reported on Hospital Compare in December 2017. Surveys are from patients discharged between April 2016 and March 2017. Scores have been adjusted for survey mode and patient-mix.

[1]The **"Top-box"** is the most positive response to HCAHPS survey items. Percentiles indicate how often patients gave positive assessments of their hospital experience. *With "Top-box" scores, the higher, the better.* For example, on "Communication with Nurses," 5% of hospitals scored 90 or higher (95th percentile) in the "Top-box," while 5% scored 72 or lower (5th percentile). The median (50th percentile) score on this measure was 80.

[2]The **"Bottom-box"** summarizes the least positive responses to HCAHPS survey items. Percentiles indicate how often patients gave negative assessments of their hospital experience. *With "Bottom-box" scores, the lower, the better.* For example, on "Communication with Nurses," 5% of hospitals scored 1 or lower (5th percentile) in the "Bottom-box," while 5% scored 9 or higher (95th percentile). The median (50th percentile) score on this measure was 4.

Source: Reprinted from Centers for Medicare & Medicaid Services (2017).

colleagues (2008) found that patients' overall rating of the hospital and their willingness to recommend had strong relationships with technical performance on all medical conditions and surgical care (correlation coefficients ranging from 0.15 to 0.63; $p<.05$ for all).

Al-Amin and Makarem (2016) used the HCAHPS survey and American Hospital Association data to punctuate the important role of DPC in affecting the overall rating of hospitals through direct patient experiences. The researchers identified organizational-level factors that affect physicians' time, commitment, and incentives, which in turn affect patient experiences. Their sample consisted of 2,756 hospitals, with 25 percent receiving poor ratings from more than 6 percent of patients. In the best-performing hospitals, no patients reported that physicians "sometimes or never" communicated well, whereas 21 percent of patients in the worst-performing hospitals reported that physicians "sometimes or never" communicated well.

DISTINGUISHING FACTORS

The ratings allow consumers to see how hospitals differ on specific characteristics appearing on HCAHPS. One of the key drivers is DPC. Quigley and colleagues (2014) collected survey data from HCHAPS during 2005–2009 of 58,251 adults at a large medical group to determine the importance of five aspects of DPC to overall physician ratings by specialty.

Measures in Quigley's survey included "explains things," "listens carefully," "gives easy-to-understand instructions," "shows respect," and "spends enough time." For each of the 28 specialties in their sample, the researchers calculated partial correlations of the five communication measures, with a 0–10 overall physician rating, controlling for patient demographics. Physician showing respect was the most important aspect of communication for 23 out of 28 specialties, with a mean partial correlation (0.27, ranging from 0.07 to 0.44 across specialties) that accounted for more than four times as much variance in the overall physician rating as any other communication item.

Three of five communication items (physician showing respect, giving easy-to-understand instructions, spending enough time) varied significantly across specialties in their associations with the overall rating ($p < 0.05$), as the patterns of variation were consistent with the nature of the specialty care. For example, spending enough time was the most important communication dimension for interventional radiology ($r = 0.35$) but mattered little for infectious diseases ($r = 0.01$). Providing easy-to-understand instructions was the most important dimension for both geriatric medicine ($r = 0.26$) and pulmonary disease ($r = 0.21$) but mattered little for radiation oncology ($r = -0.02$). Showing respect was especially important for plastic surgery ($r = 0.44$) but much less so for interventional radiology ($r = 0.07$). Specialists should target the aspects of communication that are most important for that specialty.

IMPACT OF WRITTEN COMMENTS

Most of the HCAHPS ratings are unidirectional—patients rate the quality of their experience through responses to closed-ended questions—while DPC is often interactive, encompassing many of the feelings and expectations that patients have had throughout the delivery of care.

Huppertz and Smith (2014) examined the impact of handwritten comments on the HCAHPS two global outcome measures, "overall hospital rating" and "intention to recommend." Using content analysis, they categorized the narratives as "positive," "negative," "neutral," and "mixed." Regression analysis showed that negative comments significantly affect the prediction of the two global outcome measures. Coefficients for negative comments were significant for both the overall hospital rating ($p < .011$) and intent to recommend ($p < .004$) measures. The coefficients for positive, neutral, and mixed comments were not significant, indicating that these comments did not contribute more information than quantitative ratings did.

An important issue involves the perceived gap between what healthcare leaders say about the overall quality of patient care in their hospitals and what patients indicate on the HCAHPS surveys. The next section addresses this problem.

PERCEPTUAL GAP

In a study of more than 17,000 healthcare leaders in 44 states, more than 75 percent of the hospital leaders reported that quality of care was something their hospital did well (Dunn 2012). Patients responding to the HCAHPS survey, however, did not always agree. These hospitals scored in the 43rd percentile, on average, on one of HCAHPS's measures: the number of patients who gave their hospital a rating of 9 or 10 on a scale from 0 (lowest) to 10 (highest).

These same hospitals had an average score of 88.2 on the Centers for Medicare & Medicaid Services clinical process-of-care measures. Hospitals with slightly less confident leadership—those with 50–74 percent of leaders who reported their institutions were "doing well"—performed better on core measures (94.0 average score). The survey found that leaders' perceptions did not always match the data, and many hospital leaders overestimated the performance of their organization. The gap between perception and reality (see exhibit 21.2) highlights the importance of using objective data to drive and monitor performance improvement rather than merely relying on perceptions. To reduce the gap, hospital leaders can consider the link between communication goals (e.g., responsiveness of hospital staff, pain management, communication about medicines) and outcomes (e.g., increased adherence and compliance, readmission, healthcare delivery costs, overall hospital ratings). They can also monitor the patient experience (exhibit 21.3).

Healthcare leaders must be mindful that these measures also come with significant disadvantages, such as the difficulty patients have in assessing technical aspects of care. Patients' general mood or response tendencies may also affect their evaluations.

Exhibit 21.2: Perceptual Gap

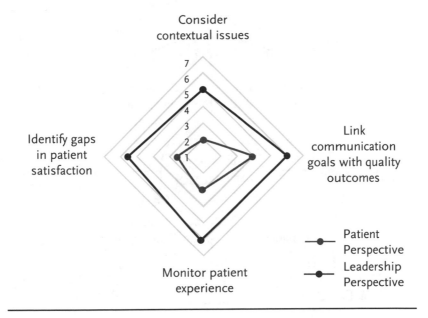

It is important to consider the interrelationships of the four domains of action holistically, as complementary undertakings. The model in exhibit 21.3 provides some assurances that parts of the system will not have to compensate for the failings of others (Belasen, Eisenberg, and Huppertz 2015).

When intentions and outcomes are aligned, they create a powerful medium by which healthcare leaders can evaluate the gaps between patient care measures and thresholds and mitigate contextual issues (e.g., physician ownership) or organizational or technological factors relevant for improving the patient experience. For example, better design of electronic health record systems and improved interpersonal communication can help physicians' daily practices of meaningful use and improve the overall patient experience (Shachak and Reis 2009).

Exhibit 21.3: Patient Satisfaction as an Organizing Principle

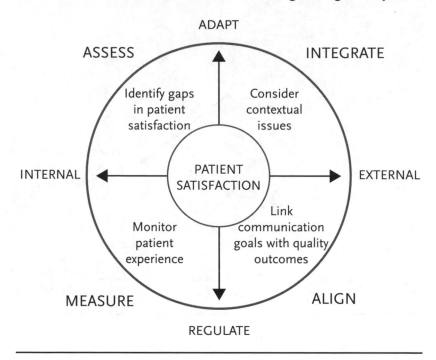

Providing consumers with useful frameworks for understanding quality helps them value the broader range of quality indicators such as safety, effectiveness, and patient centeredness.

Further, when measures are grouped into user-friendly formats, patients can see the meaning of the measures more clearly and understand how the measures relate to their personal care.

Tailoring physicians' communication style to patients' needs through informed flexibility (also called *collaborative communication*), in which caregivers seek to empower patients by removing barriers to status distinctions, is a key aspect of a successful patient-centered consultation (DuPre 2010). When this technique is accomplished, patients participate more fully and actively in the exchange and depart with an enhanced commitment to carrying out care management requirements.

Studies reported a positive relationship between patients' higher social class and doctors' level of responsiveness, as well as patients' communication styles and ability to express opinions and ask questions. Combining knowledge of the patients' background and concerns with sensitivity skills and (physician) consultative style is empowering and correlates with positive outcomes (Hall, Roter, and Katz 1988; McKinstry 2000; Street et al. 2005).

KEY TAKEAWAYS

- On a daily basis, more than 30,000 patients receive HCAHPS surveys about their recent hospital experience.
- Surveys find that many hospital leaders overestimate the performance of their organizations.
- The gap between perception and reality highlights the importance of using objective data to drive and monitor performance improvement.
- To reduce the gap, hospital leaders can consider the links between communication goals and outcomes and monitor the patient experience.
- DPC is not only important for its impact on patient outcomes but also because of its role in influencing the overall patient ratings of the hospital.
- In the best-performing hospitals, no patients reported that physicians "sometimes or never" communicated well, whereas 21 percent of patients in the worst-performing hospitals reported that physicians "sometimes or never" communicated well.
- Tailoring physicians' communication style to patients' needs through informed flexibility or collaborative communication, in which caregivers seek to empower patients by removing barriers to status distinctions, is important for a successful doctor–patient relationship.

REFERENCES

Agency for Healthcare Research and Quality. 2017. "HCAHPS Fact Sheet." Posted November 2. www.hcahpsonline.org/global assets/hcahps/facts/hcahps_fact_sheet_november_2017.pdf.

Al-Amin, M., and S. Makarem. 2016. "The Effects of Hospital-Level Factors on Patients' Ratings of Physician Communication." *Journal of Healthcare Management* 61 (1): 28–43.

Belasen, A., B. Eisenberg, and J. Huppertz. 2015. *Mastering Leadership: A Vital Resource for Healthcare Organizations.* Burlington, MA: Jones & Bartlett Learning.

Centers for Medicare & Medicaid Services. 2017. "HCAHPS Percentiles." Published December 21. www.hcahpsonline.org/ globalassets/hcahps/summary-analyses/percentiles/december -2017-public-report-april-2016---march-2017.pdf.

Clever, S. L., L. Jin, W. Levinson, and D. O. Meltzer. 2008. "Does Doctor–Patient Communication Affect Patient Satisfaction with Hospital Care? Results of an Analysis with a Novel Instrumental Variable." *Health Services Research* 43 (5): 1505–19.

Dunn, L. 2012. "6 Characteristics of High-Performing Healthcare Organizations." *Becker's Hospital Review.* www.beckershospital review.com/hospital-management-administration/6-character istics-of-high-performing-healthcare-organizations.html.

DuPre, A. 2010. *Communicating About Health: Current Issues and Perspectives*, 3rd ed. New York: Oxford University Press.

Hall, J. A., D. L. Roter, and N. R. Katz. 1988. "Meta-analysis of Correlates of Provider Behavior in Medical Encounters." *Medical Care* 26 (7): 657–75.

Health Services Advisory Group. 2019. "HCAHPS Tables on *HCAHPS On-Line*." Centers for Medicare & Medicaid Services. Modified March 27. www.hcahpsonline.org/en/ summary-analyses/#PercentileTable.

Huppertz, J., and R. Smith. 2014. "The Value of Patients' Hand-written Comments on HCAHPS Surveys." *Journal of Healthcare Management* 59 (1): 31–48.

McKinstry, B. 2000. "Do Patients Wish to Be Involved in Decision Making in the Consultation? A Cross Sectional Survey with Video Vignettes." *British Medical Journal* 321: 867–71.

Quigley, D. D., M. N. Elliott, D. O. Farley, Q. Burkhart, S. A. Skootsky, and R. D. Hays. 2014. "Specialties Differ in Which Aspects of Doctor Communication Predict Overall Physician Ratings." *Journal of General Internal Medicine* 29 (3): 447–54.

Shachak, A., and S. Reis. 2009. "The Impact of Electronic Medical Records on Patient–Doctor Communication During Consultation: A Narrative Literature Review." *Journal of Evaluation in Clinical Practice* 15 (4): 641–49.

Street, R. L., H. S. Gordon, M. Ward, E. Krupat, and R. L. Kravitz. 2005. "Patient Participation in Medical Consultations: Why Some Patients Are More Involved Than Others." *Medical Care* 43 (10): 960–69.

PART VI

Physician Leadership: Skills and Competencies

Exhibit 6: Progression of Learning

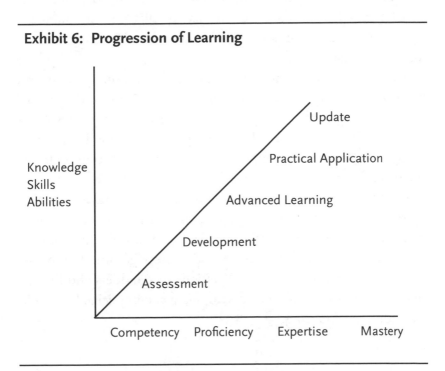

The term *manager* indicates a person in a transactional, authoritative position derived from the organizational hierarchy. A manager is concerned with internal consistency, procedures and policies, setting goals for employees, and emphasizing tasks and duties.

Conversely, a *leader* functions socially and informally, and the role is often not assigned.

One of the main differences between managers and leaders is that managers direct subordinates and leaders influence followers. However, because of the fluidity of many forms of organizational structure, managers perform leadership roles and leaders perform managerial roles. Although managers and leaders perform distinct (and often overlapping) roles, leadership is not bound by a specific hierarchical position, and practically anyone in an organization can have a leadership presence. This is especially true in healthcare organizations, where coleaders or dyads perform overlapping roles that rely heavily on effective emotional intelligence (EI) and communication competencies aimed at inspiring members and achieving high performance.

Leaders transforming healthcare exhibit visionary skills and behaviors that communicate the mission and vision of the organization and inspire new perspectives and creative ideas for resolving problems. Effective leaders have strong EI with a good balance of personality traits and use appropriate message orientations to frame the common purpose and construct the shared reality.

Chapters 22 and 23 discuss important behavioral tendencies, personality traits, and EI and use assessment instruments to demonstrate the importance of self-understanding and self-improvement. Chapters 24 and 25 introduce effective message orientations for facilitating communication with various stakeholders and for setting the stage for competency development and physician leadership education and training.

CHAPTER 22

Dyad Partners as Emotional Intelligence Leaders

INTRODUCTION

While leadership and management share similar, overlapping roles, there are also significant differences between what managers and leaders do. Management relies on control and uses its centralized authority to create structures, initiate actions, and bring order. Leadership, on the other hand, is about adapting to changing situations flexibly and effectively. Managers execute plans, follow budgets, organize the workforce, and coordinate and monitor activities. Leaders set the broader goals and align members with the vision.

The best leaders are able to control their emotions through self-awareness, self-regulation, motivation, empathy, and social skills (Goleman 1998). Emotional intelligence (EI) skills enhance your understanding of your own mood, emotions, drives, and the ability to control impulses and redirect negative attitudes toward more positive outcomes.

EMOTIONALLY INTELLIGENT LEADERS

Adaptive leaders with EI skills have the capacity to understand and manage their own emotions and the feelings of the people around them. EI skills provide leaders with a sense of integrity, which can positively affect interpersonal relationships.

Developing a high level of EI requires persistence and practice. EI leaders can quickly identify the complexities of a given situation and explain them to others. They are capable of relating well to others, building trusting relationships, reducing divergence, and establishing connections across multilevel organizational structures.

EI leaders frame the broader vision using input and feedback from all levels inside and outside the organization. Effective leaders are able to offset their own weaknesses by recruiting fellow employees who can complement their strengths.

Enhancing one's EI is a lifelong process, not an overnight panacea. It would be unrealistic to expect a quality leader to drop all his obligations and responsibilities to develop his emotional intelligence. Successful leaders improve their emotional intelligence continuously while simultaneously maintaining their personal, professional, and social lives (Belasen 2017). Emotionally intelligent leaders cannot be self-absorbed or focus solely on themselves. They still have a commitment to their organization. They need to ask the right questions, creating emotional bonds and social harmony. They balance what needs to be done with what is right for the health system. They devise plans in consultation with others and use EI skills to generate the moral commitment of individuals and groups to implementing the plans.

ASSESSING YOUR EMOTIONAL INTELLIGENCE SKILLS

In *Why Should Anyone Be Led by You*, Robert Goffee and Gareth Jones (2006) suggest that EI leaders share four common qualities: they (1) selectively show their weaknesses, (2) rely heavily on intuition to gauge the appropriate timing and display clear commitment to course of their actions, (3) manage employees with tough empathy, and (4) reveal their differences.

Verbalizing personal vulnerabilities demonstrates humility and honesty. It conveys confidence. When a leader admits to weaknesses, it creates trust and a collaborative atmosphere, which promotes unity among followers and leaders.

The ability to collect and interpret relevant data requires intuition and analysis. Much information reaches leaders from multiple directions, creating complexity and unstructured decision situations. Intuition helps reduce complexity and narrow down the available options, which can then be analyzed in a logical way. The reverse is true, too—a rational analysis may reveal a few options good enough to solve the problems, and intuition is needed to single out the right one.

Practicing tough empathy, however, requires the leader to make unpopular decisions. It prevents followers from becoming too complacent.

Revealing personal differences requires a strong sense of personal integrity and moral courage. Effective EI leaders use their differences to keep a social distance but, at the same time, make sure not to over-differentiate to avoid the perception of being arrogant.

EI leaders may acknowledge their weaknesses and vulnerabilities, but if a weakness involves incompetency, it may have an adverse effect on peers and followers. This is where assessment and development becomes indispensable. Exhibit 22.1, for example, shows how survey data reveal the gaps between current levels of beliefs and attitudes versus desired levels across the five components of EI. The next sections discuss the process of identifying those gaps.

METHODOLOGY

Assessing your EI skills, personality traits, and message orientations and learning how to adjust your relationships with others to

Exhibit 22.1: Diagnosing and Analyzing EI Skills

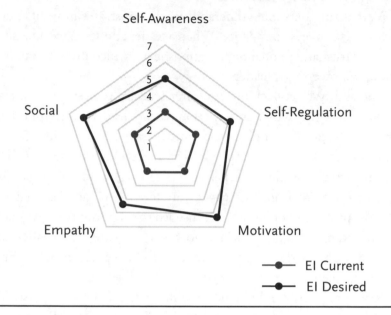

accommodate transitions in the hospital environment could help boost mutual trust and personal credibility. The survey methodology for measuring EI skills appears in exhibit 22.2.

Great leaders are aware of their own leadership style. Knowing your EI strengths and weaknesses helps reduce stress and promote healthy relationships. Improving your EI skills across the five components will make you a leader with the empathy and communication sensitivity to lead teams effectively.

Moving meaningfully from the current EI skills in exhibit 22.1 to the more desired level makes sense. Strong EI skills across the five categories facilitate positive interactions, build trust, and enhance communication and listening. Leaders make decisions that are more thoughtful and accountable. These leaders are authentic.

Exhibit 22.2: Measuring Your EI Strengths and Weaknesses

Frequency Level (Seven-Point Likert Scale)
Thinking about your attitudes and beliefs when working with teams and individuals in your healthcare system, reflect on each statement by indicating the response that best matches your beliefs, first in terms of the actual (i.e., current beliefs, expectations, views, behaviors) and then desired.

1 — *Very untrue of what I believe*
2 — *Untrue of what I believe*
3 — *Somewhat untrue of what I believe*
4 — *Neutral*
5 — *Somewhat true of what I believe*
6 — *True of what I believe*
7 — *Very true of what I believe*

Emotional Intelligence Skills	Actual	Desired
SELF-AWARENESS		
1. I recognize immediately when I am short-tempered.		
2. I am aware when I am happy.		
3. I know when I feel stressed out.		
4. I can tell when I am emotional.		
5. I am aware when I feel anxious.		
6. I can detect my own anger.		
AVG		
Self-Regulation		
7. I can let go of my anger when someone hurts my feelings.		
8. I can control my mood.		
9. I do not hold a grudge when someone annoys me.		
10. I can consciously alter my frame of mind.		
11. I do not let stressful situations overcome me.		
12. I can separate work stressors from my life.		
AVG		

(continued)

Exhibit 22.2: Measuring Your EI Strengths and Weaknesses *(continued)*

Motivation
13. I am internally motivated to accomplish challenging tasks.
14. I am motivated to complete my work on time.
15. I always meet my personal goals.
16. I set my priorities and manage my time productively.
17. I can challenge myself to accomplish difficult tasks.
18. I feel motivated when challenged.
AVG

Empathy
19. I am able to understand the other person's perspectives.
20. I can empathize with others.
21. I can tell if someone is upset with me.
22. I can understand if I am being unreasonable.
23. I can understand the effects of my decisions on others.
24. I can see things from others' point of view.
AVG

Social
25. I am a good listener when others communicate with me.
26. I do not interrupt others' conversations.
27. I enjoy interacting with others.
28. I am comfortable working with individuals and teams.
29. I am good at reconciling differences with others.
30. I know how to build respect through trust.
AVG

KEY TAKEAWAYS

- Developing strong EI skills requires persistence and practice.
- Enhancing your skills will help increase your credibility because you will focus on treating employees with empathy and respect.
- You will understand the advantage of asking the right questions in decision-making and in social settings and have a good awareness of employees' EI abilities in addition to your own.
- EI leaders can quickly identify the complexities of a given situation and explain them to others.
- Effective leaders are able to offset their own weaknesses by delegating or recruiting members who can complement their strengths.

REFERENCES

Belasen, A. 2017. *Women in Management: A Framework for Sustainable Work–Life Integration*. New York: Routledge.

Goffee, R., and G. Jones. 2006. *Why Should Anyone Be Led by You? What It Takes to Be an Authentic Leader*. Boston: Harvard Business School Press.

Goleman, D. 1998. "What Makes a Leader?" *Harvard Business Review* 76 (6): 93–102.

CHAPTER 23

Personality Traits

INTRODUCTION

Personality assessment facilitates an understanding of your strengths and weaknesses. It creates the self-awareness indispensable for self-improvement. In a dyad situation, it helps inform the partners how well they complement each other cognitively and behaviorally. The CrossTraits model, developed by Dr. Nancy Frank, is an assessment based on the five-factor model and correlated with the competing values framework (Belasen and Frank 2008). Chapter 23 explores the traits, domains of action, and leadership roles of dyads.

Relating traits to dyad leadership roles is important, because mismatches can be treated as opportunities for improvement and further development. Physicians may find that they need to adapt their personality traits situationally to meet the demands of the changing task environment.

CROSSTRAITS

Many of the dimensions and underlying assumptions of the Cross-Traits model are consistent with the frameworks presented in this book and therefore with the dyad leadership roles and domains of action (see exhibit 23.1). The four traits that make up the model include openness to experience, conscientiousness, extroversion, and agreeableness.

Exhibit 23.1: Traits Associated with Dyad Roles

Personality Traits	Domains of Action	Dyad Roles
Openness to new ideas	Innovation	Health innovator
Assertiveness	Promotion	Value strategist
Conscientiousness	Integration	Clinical integration champion
Agreeableness	Collaboration	Patient advocate

Your scores across the four domains and the resulting chart are not an indication of your performance, competency, or commitment. Instead, the chart and scores are more like an exercise in discovering values. They are useful for physicians and administrators wishing to identify strengths and weaknesses in an effort to ensure progression and achievement of learning goals. They can alert physicians and executives to areas that need to be remedied or traits that generate negative energy or convey excess. The survey appears in exhibit 23.2, with examples in exhibits 23.4–23.7.

STRESS AND TRAIT EXTREMES

Leaders sometimes exhibit extreme versions of these traits as a result of stressful challenges associated with transitions, workload pressure, time urgency, uncertainty, or unachievable goals. Some executives respond by laying low or staying away, while others resort to hyper-effective behaviors (Belasen and Belasen 2016).

As exhibit 23.3 illustrates, there is an inverse relationship between job stress and job performance. Examples of excess include rigidity and disagreeability, carelessness, timidity, and headstrongness or lack of openness.

Trait extremes are perceived by others negatively and often lead to mistrust and lack of confidence in the ability of leaders to meet stated objectives. Leaders fail to deliver when they experience the following:

- Troubled interpersonal relationships (not agreeable)
- Inability to meet objectives (not conscientious)
- Difficulty leading teams and work units (not assertive)
- Absence of behavioral flexibility (not open to new ideas)

Exhibit 23.2: Personality Assessment Questionnaire

I would describe myself as . . . (1 lowest, 5 highest)		
Traits	**Characteristics**	**Ratings**
Open	Adventurous	
	Innovative	
	Adapts well	
	Enterprising	
	AVG	
Assertive	Talkative	
	Extroverted	
	Outgoing	
	Take charge	
	AVG	
Conscientious	Detail oriented	
	Industrious	
	Precise	
	Logical	
	AVG	
Agreeable	Good-natured	
	Friendly	
	Cooperative	
	Accommodating	
	AVG	

Exhibit 23.3: Effects of Stress on Performance

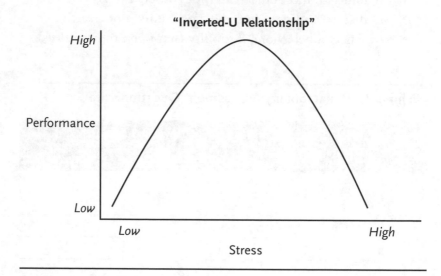

Personal weaknesses tend to magnify stress, a dynamic condition that relates to an outcome that is perceived to be important—yet unachievable, uncertain, or constrained. While low-to-moderate levels of stress stimulate the body and increase its ability to react (stimulating release of adrenaline), excessive levels of stress might lead to increased cardiovascular reactivity.

Long-term stress tends to wear people out; drain energy; and trigger detachment, burnout, and avoidance. The examples in exhibits 23.4–23.7 represent imbalances that need to be recognized and remedied.

How to Become a Better Leader

In general, aspiring leaders need to become aware of their outlier tendencies and learn how they are perceived by others. Passion, hard work and intensity are vital traits for leaders, but those same traits can also be overwhelming. The lesson here is straightforward: The bundle of traits that work for you as a leader right now can become a source of problems on short notice.

—Ginka Toegel and Jean-Louis Barsoux (2012)

OPENNESS

Being open to new ideas is a great asset for managing and leading change. It allows the leader to broaden the scope of alternatives and implement the strategy with the best chances of surviving pushback or resistance. Openness is associated with behavioral flexibility, permeability, and resilience. Too much creativity or excess of innovative thinking—with one compelling idea followed by another compelling idea, and another, and so on—may lead to a perception of the leader as a disorganized external or a great abstract thinker but one without the ability to achieve closure.

Excess in this quadrant is often the result of perfectionism and the constant need to look for or experiment with more ideas (see exhibit 23.4). Too much abstract thinking creates unnecessary complexity; it is confusing and distracting. One remedy is to take some clues from others and understand when less-than-perfect ideas are the most practical.

Exhibit 23.4: Excess Openness

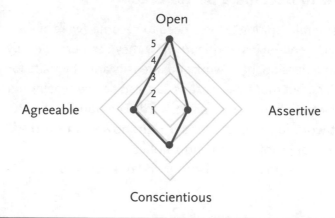

Avoid the tendency to let perfectionist paralysis stand in the way of bringing closure or stifling your team's creativity. Encourage mistakes and risks in your workplace by drawing on other quadrants or by shifting some of your excess energy from change and adaptation to stability and control. Increase your attention to the opposite trait by becoming more conscientious. Shift sideways by reducing ambiguity (becoming more assertive) and by communicating realistic ideas and options more clearly (becoming more agreeable).

ASSERTIVENESS

Leadership is a process of influence and involves the ability to shape the attitudes of followers. Leaders that push their influence to the extreme (e.g., forcing the issue, insisting on being in charge, withholding or holding up information) are vocal, authoritative, and opinionated.

These leaders are disrespectful of others' viewpoints and have domineering attitudes.

They are distrusted until they prove themselves trustworthy and often are perceived by followers as ineffective. Excessive assertiveness is demonstrated by monopolizing airtime during team meetings, dominating the narratives, and not listening to others.

It is quite conceivable that by simply listening more, agreeing with others, and paying more attention to others' ideas and alternatives, you can mitigate your assertiveness level. Avoid the tendency to define problems in terms of proposed solutions. Asking the right questions rather than prescribing solutions is a great adjustment that can help shift the profile in exhibit 23.5 more toward the center.

CONSCIENTIOUSNESS

Conscientiousness reflects structure and discipline, formal logic, efficiency, and attention to detail. The conscientious leader prefers to follow rules and embrace the status quo. Excess in this quadrant might create the perception that you are an obsessive monitor who tends to micromanage people and processes.

Exhibit 23.5: Excess Assertiveness

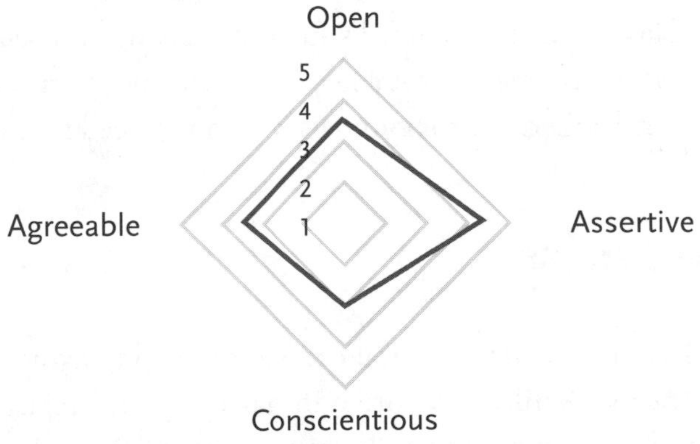

Open

5
4
3
2
1

Agreeable

Assertive

Conscientious

Exhibit 23.6: Excess Conscientiousness

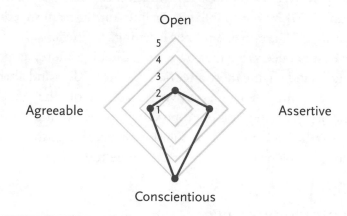

While being conscientious may get you the results you expect, in the long run it is a losing proposition, as followers and peers may resent your style or switch to questioning the validity of your assumptions (see exhibit 23.6). Micromanagers risk disempowering their followers, which increases the risk of burnout and reduces employees' confidence and trust.

A simple remedy is to balance the tendencies of this quadrant toward control and detail orientation with openness (opposite quadrant), engagement (adjacent quadrant), and agreeableness (adjacent quadrant). Playing the role of devil's advocate (asking yourself, "What if . . . ?") may help balance your need for control, attention to the micro level, and adherence to boundaries with the need for flexibility.

AGREEABLENESS

Agreeable leaders who use this trait excessively tend to avoid conflicts and disruptions. While they thrive in harmony and relationships, they often appear weak and vulnerable. This is true when agreeableness is extreme—to the point where the leader is perceived as permissive and afraid of confrontation (see exhibit 23.7). Under

Exhibit 23.7: Excess Agreeableness

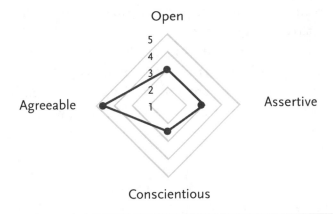

these conditions, followers may perceive you as less confident and unassertive, someone who often cannot be trusted in times of crises. One way to mitigate these perceptions is to become more assertive or competitive (qualities associated with the opposite trait).

Balancing the expectations of this quadrant with the demands in the other quadrants can help bring more structure and clarity and generate better ideas for solving problems. Practicing situational leadership (knowing when to intervene and when to let go) is a great way to reduce the effects of excess in this quadrant and to balance individual considerations with a task orientation.

KEY TAKEAWAYS

- Personality assessment facilitates an understanding of your strengths and weaknesses and provides a powerful insight into a leader's learning curve.
- The association of traits with the dyad leadership roles is important, as mismatches can be viewed as opportunities for further learning and self-improvement.

- Self-assessment and a greater understanding of the personalities of dyad leaders can alert physicians and executives to areas that require remedy or traits that trigger negative energy or convey excess.
- Excess includes headstrongness (lack of openness), timidity (lack of assertiveness), carelessness (lack of conscientiousness), and inflexibility (lack of agreeability).
- Practicing situational leadership (knowing when to intervene and when to let go) is a great way to reduce the effects of excess.

REFERENCES

Belasen, A. T., and A. R. Belasen. 2016. "Value in the Middle: Cultivating Middle Managers in Healthcare Organizations." *Journal of Management Development* 35 (9): 1149–62.

Belasen, A., and N. Frank. 2008. "Competing Values Leadership: Quadrant Roles and Personality Traits." *Leadership and Organization Development Journal* 29 (2): 127–43.

Toegel, G., and J. L. Barsoux. 2012. "How to Become a Better Leader." *MIT Sloan Management Review* 53 (3): 51–60.

CHAPTER 24

Message Orientation

INTRODUCTION

Communication is the vibrant thread that ties together employee vitality, organizational clarity of direction and purpose, and the results and progress of both. Dyad leaders use communication as a tool to achieve health system goals. However, leaders must communicate carefully to achieve positive outcomes, not merely to fill the silence. In fact, overcommunicating can be as destructive as undercommunicating. The former can cause confusion, misunderstanding, and loss of productivity, and it can overwhelm those on the receiving end. The latter can lead to distrust, uncertainty, low morale, and a lack of alignment.

How managers can select the right tone to communicate different tasks and goals, and how they can find the most effective message orientation for each task or goal, is an important question. This chapter demonstrates the importance of aligning message orientations to the type of stakeholders that dyad leaders engage in their daily operations. It includes a self-assessment survey to help identify personal strengths and weaknesses.

COMMUNICATION PERSPECTIVES

Often managers at different levels see themselves as members of separate constituencies rather than as members of the same team in the same organization. The common language offered by the competing values framework (CVF) ameliorates this separation—it is essentially an organizational language that is used to identify performance criteria that are common across the hierarchy. The following passages explain.

Communication from a transactional perspective is largely information based and downward directed (from management to employees). Clear, concise, targeted instructions to employees lead to the accomplishment of tasks that fuel results. Communication from a transformational perspective is largely vision based and multi-directional—it moves upward and downward, as well as laterally. But how can managers select the right dyad role to communicate different tasks and goals and use the most effective message orientation for each task or situation?

Clarifying dyad roles and expectations can help minimize role ambiguity and reduce the potential for role conflict. Likewise, interpersonal conflicts associated with turf issues, status, and power dynamics may be avoided in favor of developing a constructive dialogue and encouraging positive communication.

MESSAGE ORIENTATIONS AND DYAD ROLES

Rogers and Hildebrandt (1993) and Belasen (2008) suggest that each quadrant in the CVF represents a different message orientation (emphasizing style over content) with significant parallels and polar opposites: relational, promotional, transformational, and hierarchical (see exhibit 24.1).

Relational messages are aimed at personal relationships, informal interactions, peer communications, and maintaining an awareness of

Exhibit 24.1: Message Orientations

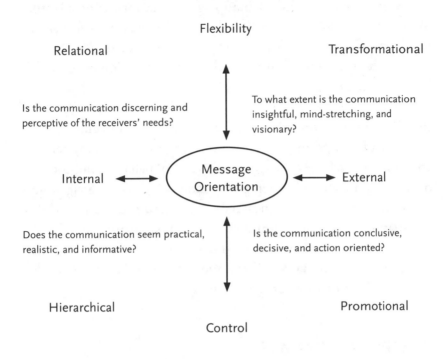

the importance of the individual's role in completing the organization's mission. When dyad leaders function in the patient advocate role, for example, they rely on a relational approach to communication that places emphasis on patients' insights and feedback. They focus on social identity, common understandings, commitment, and concerns for human development.

A promotional orientation fits the behaviors displayed by the value strategist, who relies on persuasion strategies to meet hospital objectives. Promotional messages relate to the mission of the organization in its efforts to meet external expectations for health services, to perform productively in order to maximize returns on equity, and to enhance performance credibility and organizational accountability.

Transformational messages match the styles and behaviors of the health innovator, who excels in selling ideas effectively and meeting future organizational and adaptation goals. She focuses on adapting to new market requirements, branding, and reputation management to address the interests of external stakeholders. Success is determined by the extent to which framing of the communication is insightful, horizon expanding, and visionary.

Hierarchical message orientations, on the other hand, align with the clinical integration champion who focuses on integrating individuals and groups through work processes, metrics, and systems of control. Hierarchical messages reflect rules of behavior and codified decisions aimed at regularizing interactions between managers and employees. Hierarchical messages characterize the flow and dissemination of formal communications across organizational lines. Success is determined by whether the communication seems realistic, practical, and informative. These orientations and examples of different applications appear in exhibit 24.2.

COMPETING FRAMES

Recognizing the existence of competing frames becomes a powerful personal roadmap for self-improvement (i.e., diagramming personal profiles)—a tool to help dyads understand how well they need to balance the different orientations across the quadrants and the steps they can take for improving oral and written communication.

CREATING YOUR OWN MESSAGE-ORIENTATION PROFILE

Exhibit 24.3 is a survey about your communication approach. For each question, indicate the behavior that you will most likely use.

Exhibit 24.2: Matching Message Orientations to Different Constituencies

Relational	Transformational
Purpose: Establishing integrity, rapport, trust, confidence, and commitment **Medium and tone:** Conversational, honest, committed, personal, supportive, evocative; full of familiar words, inclusive pronouns; reinforces feedback **Focus:** Receiver centered **Audience:** Employees **Example:** Informal chats, cafeteria talks, reflective listening	**Purpose:** Challenging receivers to accept horizon-expanding vision **Medium and tone:** Visionary, charismatic, vivid, enthusiastic, emphatic; employing colorful metaphors, symbols, and oral delivery or unorthodox written communication **Focus:** Idea centered, futuristic, and rhetorical **Audience:** Customers, investors **Example:** CEO speech, written strategic plan, smart talk, communicating vision
Hierarchical	**Promotional**
Purpose: Providing clear directions to receivers **Medium and tone:** Neutral, precise words, controlled, sequential, factually accurate; using standard constructions, structural rigor, logical progression, realistic presentation, conventional documents, concrete examples, lists, tables, and audit reports **Focus:** Communication-channel centered **Audience:** Regulators **Example:** Policy statements, procedural specifications, rules, standards, written documents, computer printouts, unaddressed letters, memos, directives	**Purpose:** Promoting an idea, selling a product or service, persuading receivers, establishing credibility **Medium and tone:** Decisive, engaging, original, assertive, declarative, prepositional; employing vivid examples and credible evidence; engendering a sense of urgency **Focus:** Argument centered **Audience:** Partners, stakeholders **Example:** Sales presentations, recommendations to senior managers, press releases, directives, quarterly results, financial reports

You will mark two responses: one to describe your messages as they are now, another to describe messages as you wish they were. These responses will be the same if the message is exactly as you think it should be for the situation.

Exhibit 24.3: Survey Methodology for Measuring Message Orientations

Frequency Level (Seven-Point Likert Scale)
Next to each statement indicate the response that best matches your situation.

1 — *Never*
2 — *Rarely (in fewer than 10 percent of my chances)*
3 — *Occasionally (in about 30 percent of my chances)*
4 — *Sometimes (in about 50 percent of my chances)*
5 — *Frequently (in about 70 percent of my chances)*
6 — *Usually (in about 90 percent of my chances)*
7 — *Every time*

	Actual	Desired
1. When I communicate new directions, I make sure that I am discerning and perceptive of the receivers' reactions. [**aware**]		
2. When asked for my opinion, the tone of my messages is forceful and prevailing. [**emphatic**]		
3. I inspire peers or team members with messages that are horizon-expanding and visionary. [**insightful**]		
4. I encourage communications that are creative and original. [**innovative**]		
5. My messages are interesting and stimulating. [**engaging**]		
6. I am conclusive and decisive when I communicate goals to team members. [**action oriented**]		
7. I make big efforts to use realistic and informative messages. [**practical**]		
8. My statements and messages are focused and logical. [**organized**]		
9. I use rigor and consistency in communicating with peers. [**precise**]		

(continued)

10. I make sure that my messages are technically correct. [**accurate**]

11. I use credible and believable communications with peers and team members. [**plausible**]

12. My communications with others are open and candid. [**honest**]

In this example (exhibit 24.4), the manager seems to place more weight on promotional and hierarchical message orientations than on transformational and lateral styles, suggesting a preference to work with individuals within boundaries of trust, structures, and rules. This manager's profile, however, seems to deflect the need for placing equal value on the upper side of the framework, where messages are aimed at generating new ideas and a commitment to engage in positive communications. When patients, employees, peers, and supervisors provide their inputs, this framework can become a powerful tool for guiding improvement efforts based on expectations from others.

THE ADVANTAGE OF CREATING APPROPRIATE MESSAGES

Dyads can gain a number of advantages by using the model of message orientations for identifying their strengths and weaknesses and by taking steps to improve the effectiveness of their communication profiles. They can also use the relative strengths of the partners to the dyad to complement each other's predominant orientations. Having a strong understanding of the frequency (number of times), subject (whom the message is directed to), and the tenacity (power of the message or the source of the message) of the message can

Exhibit 24.4: Current and Desired Message Orientations

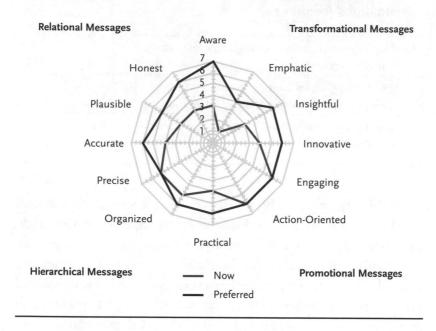

help mitigate communication roadblocks, clarifying organizational directions and expectations.

The model is particularly relevant for explaining communications and message orientations in transitioning healthcare organizations. Knowing in advance what managers communicate, as well as detecting the tone of the messages, should help peers and direct reports avoid second-guessing the importance of objectives and instructions, consistent with the expectations of top executives and directors.

When the lines of communication are clear and the messages reach their target audiences with appropriate orientation, the consistency of organizational communication increases. This should also help reduce the opportunity for miscommunication and the potential for conflict between senders and receivers. Knowing that managers at all levels of the organization are aware of the four orientations provides an additional tool for developing a common language across administrative levels for sharing expectations. Awareness of these differences could help ameliorate unnecessary frustrations and misunderstandings among managers (Belasen and Frank 2010). When used by dyad leaders, these message orientations provide an avenue for engaging employees in such a way that optimal performance becomes possible.

KEY TAKEAWAYS

- Communication from a transactional perspective is largely information based and downward directed.
- Communication from a transformational perspective is largely vision based and multidirectional—it flows upward, downward, and laterally.
- Recognizing the existence of competing frames becomes a powerful personal roadmap for self-improvement and can function as a tool to help dyads balance different orientations and improve oral and written communication.
- Dyad leaders can also use the complementary strengths of the partners to align messages to stakeholders.

REFERENCES

Belasen, A. T. 2008. *The Theory and Practice of Corporate Communication: A Competing Values Perspective.* Thousand Oaks, CA: Sage Publications.

Belasen, A., and N. Frank. 2010. "A Peek Through the Lens of the Competing Values Framework: What Managers Communicate and How." *Atlantic Journal of Communication* 18 (5): 280–96.

Rogers, P. S., and H. W. Hildebrandt. 1993. "Competing Values Instruments for Analyzing Written and Spoken Management Messages." *Human Resource Management Journal* 32 (1): 121–42.

CHAPTER 25

Competency Development

INTRODUCTION

Healthcare executives, who often do not possess a concrete understanding of the clinical environment, often fail to recognize how physicians think, decide, and act. While the supervisory structure through which leaders rise operates through pyramidal reporting relationships, clinical leaders rely on a collegial orientation and a focus on the patient or service interface.

The Case for Physician Leaders

Traditional leadership is morphing from a top-down approach to one that is more matrixed and collaborative. Where traditional leadership was more paternalistic, with leaders crafting a vision, delineating specific performance goals, and focusing the team on the work arena, leaders of today work to inspire performance, employ emotional intelligence, empower and motivate their workers, and help team members strike a balance between work and home.
—American Hospital Association (2014)

The dyad, which pairs an administrator with a physician partner, creates a powerful learning model that reinforces the movement of physicians from one stage of development to another, depending on scope and range of responsibilities. These stages reflect a progressive movement on the dyad administrative ladder and the pertinent skills essential in each stage: technical, interpersonal, and strategic. The dyad, therefore, is congruent with the growth strategy of an integrated health system—from management bound by discipline toward management across disciplines.

STAGES OF DEVELOPMENT

As exhibit 25.1 shows, aspiring physician leaders—those with the capacity to move beyond their clinical task environment to lead and manage individuals, teams, or service lines—often transition through three important stages of skill building. Technical tasks are linked to the clinical discipline, specialized knowledge, and compliance. Interpersonal tasks involve leading, motivating, and cultivating direct reports. Strategic tasks are associated with financial reports, analysis, and strategic communication, including direct involvement in headquarter projects and boardroom discussions. As physicians progress along the leadership pathway, the need for developing leadership and management skills and competencies to match the new task environment becomes a priority.

Practicing physician leaders often head a care team, medical group, or health system. If they head a care team, they are often in charge of several clinicians in a specialized unit. These team members share goals and have a common understanding of their tasks, and most of their responsibilities require technical and interpersonal skills. A medical group, however, consists of several units, committees, or projects, and typically requires physicians with some administrative experience. Interfunctional collaboration skills and some system thinking skills are vital for the success of the medical group. Systemwide operations require physicians with strong

Exhibit 25.1: Physician Leadership Development

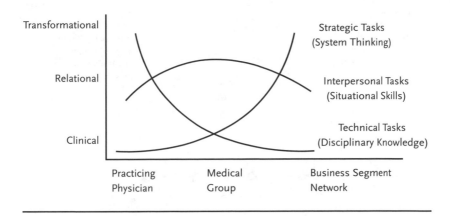

strategic skills to lead hospitals, medical groups, executives, managers, and partners. Technical expertise, interpersonal skills, and, to a large degree, conceptual strategizing and systems thinking skills are crucial for the success of the leader.

KNOWLEDGE AREAS, APPLIED MANAGEMENT, ANALYTICS, AND STRATEGY

In addition to having strong clinical knowledge, physician leaders need to have emotional intelligence (EI) and applied skills in management, analytics skills, and strategy. This range of abilities allows them to lead medical groups, supervise service lines, or manage a larger hospital system effectively. These three sets of skills are also consistent with the overall framework described in this book and reframed in exhibit 25.2 to reflect the relevant skills for the dyad roles. This framework is also consistent with the American Hospital Association (2014) leadership education core elements.

Following the path outlined in exhibit 25.1, developing self-awareness and EI skills, cultivating and promoting teamwork, and

Exhibit 25.2: Skills and Knowledge Areas

Leading Teams
Emotional Intelligence
Facilitating Change
Interpersonal Communication
Situational Leadership

Negotiation
Conflict Resolution
Business Development
External Relations
Trust Building/Credibility
Innovation and Change
  Leadership

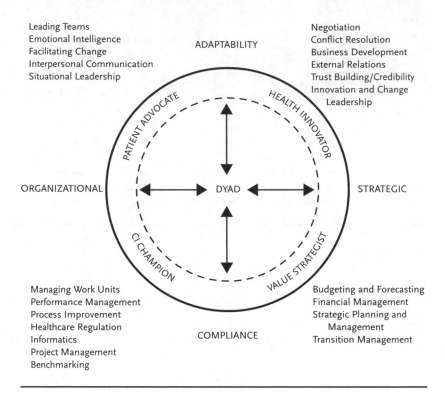

ORGANIZATIONAL

STRATEGIC

Managing Work Units
Performance Management
Process Improvement
Healthcare Regulation
Informatics
Project Management
Benchmarking

Budgeting and Forecasting
Financial Management
Strategic Planning and
  Management
Transition Management

championing interfunctional collaboration are always a good start. Moving forward, training in transition management and continuous process improvement sets the foundation for developing internal business skills. For senior executives, strategic decision-making, financial management, and economic analysis of healthcare markets shift the learning to the system level, where visioning is performed and strategic initiatives to drive change are honed.

The framework shown in exhibit 25.2 emphasizes transcending apparent contradictions at both the operational and strategic levels to identify win–win solutions. It encourages leaders to view tasks and responsibilities from a unified "both/and" perspective, rather than a binary "either/or" perspective. As a leadership development tool, the framework helps to identify strengths and weaknesses with insights about relevant training and education to meet future development demands and close potential gaps (Belasen, Eisenberg, and Huppertz 2015).

COMPETENCY DEVELOPMENT

The most effective leadership development program is experiential learning based on a competency approach supported by active mentoring and coaching. The competency approach begins with a self-assessment to identify strengths (sweet spots) and weaknesses (blind spots).

Remedying weaknesses is achieved through development (skill building), advanced learning (principles, applied knowledge), practical applications (expertise, transfer of knowledge), and updates (currency). These steps appear in exhibit 25.3. The steps of development are progressive and represent a movement toward proficiency in knowledge and skills that must be updated over time to remain current and stay abreast of changes and practices in the field of hospital management (National Institutes of Health 2009).

MENTORING

Active mentors that guide and coach the development of key physician leaders can help accelerate the progressive learning of dyad physician leaders. Mentoring is a transformational behavior that serves aspiring physician leaders well. Mentoring can go beyond a

How Top Three Health Systems Develop Physician Leaders In-House

As the business of health care becomes increasingly tied to clinical outcomes, the demand for qualified physician leaders at hospitals and health systems now far outpaces the supply. With increased competition for experienced physician executives, it is more important than ever to be able to pull from an internal pool of physician talent.

However, only 47% of health care organizations have a development pipeline for physician leaders. If you are thinking of building a leadership development program—or optimizing your own—read on to learn about three successful programs.

Baylor Scott & White's Hands-on Approach to Leadership Development

Baylor Scott & White (BSW) Health's Executive Education Program (BSWEEP) has been a proven success. . . . BSWEEP provides emerging leaders (e.g., physician and administrative supervisors, project leads, committee members) with the opportunity to employ their business knowledge and prepare for future leadership roles. . . .

BSWEEP's 13-month curriculum consists of 12 required sessions that include both course work and team-based projects. Here are the details:

- **BSWEEP coursework:** Features accounting, marketing, psychology, advocacy, leadership, and finance.
- **Team-based projects:** Six-person, multidisciplinary teams complete one BSW-specific project and several complementary exercises across each of the two semesters. Examples include: *Should we develop a Sleep Center near UMC or a Dialysis Center in Waco? What is the proper scale and timeline for constructing a new OR tower? Should we have a Mexico International Center and where should it be located?*

—Megan Zweig and Virginia Hite (2017)

one-on-one relationship; it can take shape in a group setting with peer mentoring and with reciprocal relationships in which everyone in the group is a mentor and a mentee. Mentoring might also help physicians overcome cultural barriers and tough workplace practices, challenge existing values and norms, and focus on the larger context rather than routine tasks.

A physician mentor, regardless of setting, should empower aspiring physician leaders by fostering autonomy, personal responsibility, problem solving, and decision-making skills. Effective mentoring includes sponsorship, exposure, coaching, counseling, help overcoming bureaucratic hurdles, and social support. Mentor transformational leadership also benefits the self-development and self-clarity of aspiring physicians, important influencers on efficacy and confidence. A transformational mentor can help facilitate the attainment of physician development and growth along the learning curve to mastery (see exhibit 25.3).

Exhibit 25.3: Progression of Learning

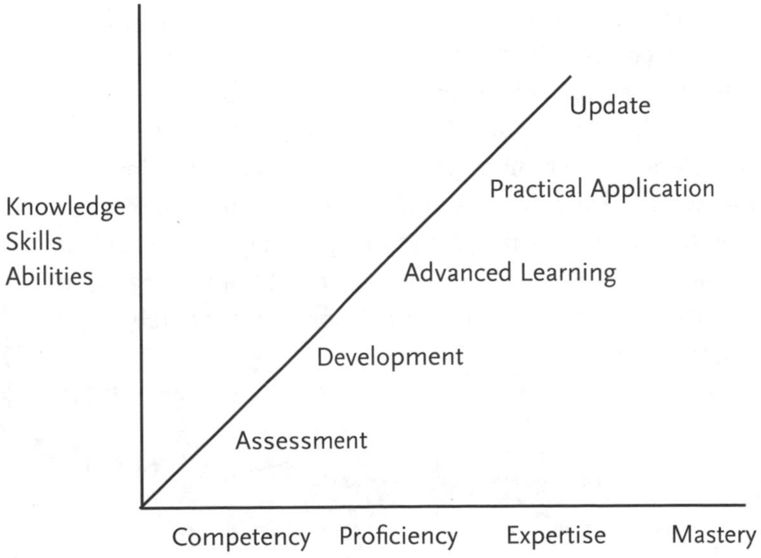

Looking to Develop Physician Leaders? Invest in Mentoring

Hospital executives looking to find leaders among their physician ranks would be wise to invest in creating and maintaining a mentorship program. Such efforts can go a long way toward improving care and lowering costs, according to an article in *Hospitals & Health Networks*.

Mentorship programs, according to Maine Medical Center CMO Peter Bates, put into practice "abstract concepts" taught in the classroom, making retention of information a much more tangible achievement. "Having a mentor to work with someone on the application of competencies . . . to a specific project is much more powerful as a learning tool than just talking about these skills," Bates says.

Designing a strong program, however, is no small feat. A recent survey conducted by the National Center for Healthcare Leadership shows that evidence-based leadership development is more successful at health systems and hospitals affiliated with systems, likely due to a larger pool of available resources.

Currently, Wisconsin-based Aurora Medical Group picks its physician leaders from management committees that supervise various departments throughout the hospital, according to *H&HN*. "By observing the thought processes and engagement levels of committee participants, we can obtain insights into which physicians have the interest, the fortitude . . . to develop into physician leaders," says Jon Kluge, vice president of clinical operations. "The management committees give physicians an opportunity to get involved in leadership and decision-making."

—Dan Bowman (2011)

KEY TAKEAWAYS

- The dyad, which pairs an administrator with a physician partner, creates a powerful learning model that reinforces the movement of physicians through a sequence of skill building and development.
- Aspiring physician leaders often transition through three important stages of skill building during their career path: EI, business analytics, and strategic leadership.
- The most effective leadership development program is experiential learning based on a competency approach and supported by active mentoring and coaching.
- Active mentors that guide and coach the development of aspiring physician leaders can help accelerate the learning curve of dyad physician leaders.

REFERENCES

American Hospital Association. 2014. "Physician Leadership Education." Accessed April 1, 2019. www.ahaphysicianforum.org/files/pdf/LeadershipEducation.pdf.

Belasen, A., B. Eisenberg, and J. Huppertz. 2015. *Mastering Leadership: A Vital Resource for Healthcare Organizations*. Burlington, MA: Jones & Bartlett Learning.

Bowman, D. 2011. "Looking to Develop Physician Leaders? Invest in Mentoring." *FierceHealthcare*. Published August 12. www.fiercehealthcare.com/healthcare/looking-to-develop-physician-leaders-invest-mentoring.

National Institutes of Health. 2009. "Competencies Proficiency Scale." Updated January 12. https://hr.nih.gov/working-nih/competencies/competencies-proficiency-scale.

Zweig, M., and V. Hite. 2017. "How Three Top Health Systems Develop Physician Leaders In-House." Advisory Board. Published March 27. www.advisory.com/research/physician-executive-council/prescription-for-change/2017/03/physician-leaders.

PART VII

Conclusion

The growing demands imposed by the shift to population health management, the accelerated rate of consolidation in the healthcare sector, and the sheer magnitude and complexity of change involving Centers for Medicare & Medicaid Services compliance costs are important factors in driving the healthcare CEO turnover rate to record highs. The rate of departure broke 20 percent for the first time in 2013 and averaged 18 percent between 2014 and 2017 (American College of Healthcare Executives 2018). Some leaders have postponed their retirement, thinking that their hospitals will be acquired soon after the ascent of a successor (Witt/Kieffer 2016).

With rising CEO turnover rates, health systems need to develop adequate succession programs to identify and train new leaders. Moreover, these programs should include a robust talent pipeline with an emphasis on appropriate selection and development strategies (Belasen and Belasen 2016). The pipeline should also have a strong physician leadership presence based on an "interdisciplinary structure that supports collaboration in decision-making between physicians and hospital executives" (American Hospital Association 2015).

The chapters in this book examined the evolving roles of executive leadership in hospitals and integrated health systems and reviewed successful forms of complementary leadership (or dyad) to help close the gaps in hospital leadership.

The concluding chapter anchors the expanded role of integrated physician–hospital leadership in learning and mentoring. It highlights the importance of having clinical competence as well as mastering the executive leadership and interaction skills to deal with emerging goals and needs. Developing physician leaders is paramount to the success of integrated health systems.

REFERENCES

American College of Healthcare Executives. 2018. "Hospital CEO Turnover Rate Remains Steady." Published June 14. www.ache.org/learning-center/research/about-ceos/hospital -ceo-turnover-rate-2017.

American Hospital Association. 2015. "Integrated Leadership for Hospitals and Health Systems: Principles for Success." Accessed April 3. www.aha.org/system/files/2018-01/ ahaamaintegrleadership.pdf.

Belasen, A. T., and A. R. Belasen. 2016. "Value in the Middle: Cultivating Middle Managers in Healthcare Organizations." *Journal of Management Development* 35 (9): 1149–62.

Witt/Kieffer. 2016. *Executive Succession and Transition in Healthcare: A Collection of Best Practices from Witt/Kieffer.* Accessed April 1, 2019. www.wittkieffer.com/file/thought-leadership/ secure-downloads/Executive%20Succession_and_Transition _in_Healthcare_electronic.pdf.

CHAPTER 26

Sustaining the Dyad

REALIGNMENT

With rising CEO turnover rates in the healthcare sector, health systems need to develop adequate succession programs to identify and train new leaders. Moreover, these programs should build a strong talent pipeline for those already working in the organization, especially since it costs less to develop and retain a cadre of leaders in-house than to hire and retrain new managers.

However, various leadership development programs typically draw on traditional approaches that fit stable and predictable environments. These approaches are inappropriate for handling the complexity of healthcare. The famous adage "we cannot solve our problems with the same level of thinking that created them" is instructive when it comes to understanding the leadership challenges in the current healthcare environment. Historically, hospitals have been slow to adapt to change and implement innovation in multi-specialty groups, which have subcultures that are less collegial and lower levels of organizational identity and trust.

Traditional hospital management, with silos and top-down executive oversight that aligns with relatively predictable healthcare delivery, is no longer a good fit with the integrated strategy of health systems. The complex nature of healthcare delivery depends on multiple interdependent parties, contradictory expectations, and volatile regulatory environments. It is also characterized by evolving pay structures and patient care requirements that are fundamentally different from typical business-to-business or business–consumer relationships. In these hospitals, executive decisions—be they financial, human resource-related, or concerning service delivery—are often made separate from the context of how care is provided.

While clinical and nonclinical personnel share the responsibility for patient goals and patient care, executive decisions are mostly administrative or isolated from points of impact. As a result, the chances for faulty decisions and unintended consequences in traditional forms of leadership are much greater.

COMPLEXITY AND THE DYAD STRUCTURE

Understanding and managing the complexity of healthcare requires leaders with strengths that reflect administrative and emotional intelligence (EI) skills, as well as clinical and financial performance abilities. However, relatively few leadership development programs address EI, personal growth, or self-awareness. The outcomes of clinical integration could be greatly enhanced through effective development of teamwork and social skills. However, current processes of selecting and training physicians often emphasize the myth of the heroic lone healer, minimizing doctors' ability to develop collaborative skills (Morse 2010). Instead, the focus of leadership development programs should be on paired leadership structures, or dyads, that engage physicians and administrators, not just the internal hierarchy.

To succeed, health systems must become quality centered, safe, streamlined, measured, evidence based, value driven, innovative, fair, equitable, and physician led (Angood and Birk 2014). Making physicians an integral part of hospital leadership makes sense. The co-leadership structure of the dyad helps to transition physicians to important leadership positions in transforming health systems. The dyad model mitigates the constraints of the disciplinary structure, improves the way clinical and business leaders work together, and optimizes the value of coordinated care.

A generic approach to leadership development cannot capture the dynamics and often-contradictory demands of healthcare environments, whether they are internal or external. Responding to simultaneous pressures from partners and regulators necessitates strong adaptation and performance management skills, while adhering to community needs and improving patient care require strong empathy and communication skills. When aligned with organizational goals, effective leadership development in health systems helps sustain a pipeline of capable leaders and prepare them for executive and board positions.

RELEVANCE AND ACCOUNTABILITY

When asked why doctors make good hospital managers, Cleveland Clinic CEO Delos "Toby" Cosgrove, MD, immediately answered, "Peer-to-peer credibility." Clinicians are more inclined to trust a leader whose initial experience provides direct knowledge and insight into their challenges, motivations, and desire to have patient-focused approach (Stoller, Goodall, and Baker 2016). In addition, studies have shown that 69 percent of physician leaders agree that doctors should be accountable for costs, as well as quality of care (Navigant 2015).

According to the Physicians Advocacy Institute (PAI), in 2015, 25 percent of medical practices were owned by a hospital or health system. Hospitals employed 38 percent of all US physicians, a 50 percent increase since 2012. The number of employed physicians totaled 95,000 in 2012. By 2015, there were more than 140,000, and by mid-2016, physician employment had grown an additional 11 percent. During that period, hospitals acquired 5,000 physician practices. PAI's study underscores the continued trend toward physician employment, part of the larger movement toward consolidation in the healthcare system (PAI 2019, 2016).

In 2016, the Centers for Medicare & Medicaid Services also reported that physician-led accountable care organizations, as well as those constituted by a physician–hospital partnership, were more likely to improve quality and lower cost enough to earn shared savings.

THE DYAD STRUCTURE AS A LEARNING INCUBATOR

While the dyad structure in which physicians and nonclinician managers share leadership responsibilities might appear to be less desirable to a physician-led organization, the dyad is an excellent learning experience for aspiring physician executives.

Critics of the dyad structure argue that the dyad does not go far enough to prepare doctors to be organizational leaders. Furthermore, the dyad structure provides disincentives to learn about fundamental practices of business and gain critical financial, operational, and management skills—limiting physicians' ability to grow into stronger leaders or advance further in the organization (Perry, Mobley, and Brubaker 2017). This book argues the contrary. Career development and leadership development ought to be two sides of the same coin.

When physicians with leadership potential are supported by appropriate management education and development programs and paired with seasoned administrators, learning is augmented experientially. Working side-by-side with business managers, who often serve as active mentors or role models for aspiring physician leaders, is a valuable learning experience as well. Leadership skills are sustained with experience, practice, coaching, or mentorship and leadership training.

The focus of the management education and development program should be on action learning and on preparing a platform for leadership roles that reflect the evolving challenges and organizational contexts facing physicians. Because clinical responsibilities do not always offer optimal conditions for physicians to advance administrative careers at earlier stages, the focus of leadership development programs should be on helping physicians master business knowledge and on strengthening their ability to make decisions in the broader context of integrated health systems. To be effective leaders, physicians need to shift their leadership focus from the disciplinary to systems thinking.

CLEVELAND CLINIC ACADEMY

The Cleveland Clinic has a training program called the Cleveland Clinic Academy (CCA). The course Leading in Healthcare is central to the CCA curriculum; it consists of 10 days of off-site training in leadership competencies, focusing on emotional intelligence (with 360-degree feedback and executive coaching), team building, conflict resolution, and situational leadership (Stoller, Goodall, and Baker 2016). The curriculum aligns essential skills to help prospective CCA participants identify courses by requisite competencies (Stoller 2008; Stoller, Berkowitz, and Bailin 2007; Stoller, Coulton, and Kay 2006).

Benchmarking successful leadership models, such as those seen at Cleveland Clinic or Mayo Clinic, create opportunities for physicians to be trained and hired to lead health systems in transformation. The benefits are widespread—hospital quality scores are approximately 25 percent higher in physician-run hospitals than in manager-run hospitals (Goodall 2011). Viewing the CCA competency-based curriculum through the lens of the framework developed in this book can be useful for physician development (see exhibit 26.1). The framework can help participants and curriculum designers to group and differentiate the competencies by common distinctions between management and leadership and by relevant dyad roles.

Exhibit 26.1: Aligning CCA Curriculum with Dyad Roles

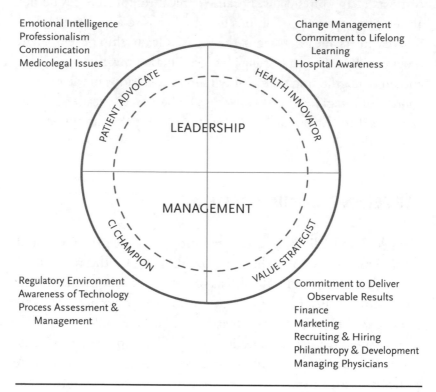

Emotional Intelligence
Professionalism
Communication
Medicolegal Issues

Change Management
Commitment to Lifelong
    Learning
Hospital Awareness

PATIENT ADVOCATE

HEALTH INNOVATOR

LEADERSHIP

MANAGEMENT

CI CHAMPION

VALUE STRATEGIST

Regulatory Environment
Awareness of Technology
Process Assessment &
    Management

Commitment to Deliver
    Observable Results
Finance
Marketing
Recruiting & Hiring
Philanthropy & Development
Managing Physicians

Moreover, the framework can help participants in leadership development programs identify relative strengths and weaknesses and select degree programs, courses, graduate certificates, or workshops to remedy weaknesses and use training and development to close potential gaps. One example appears in exhibit 26.2. Participants can prioritize the direction of the training and development by selecting areas with the greatest potential to improve their learning curve. Three examples of the gaps between the actual and desired levels of training include awareness of technology, managing physicians, and recruiting and hiring.

Exhibit 26.2: Gap Analysis

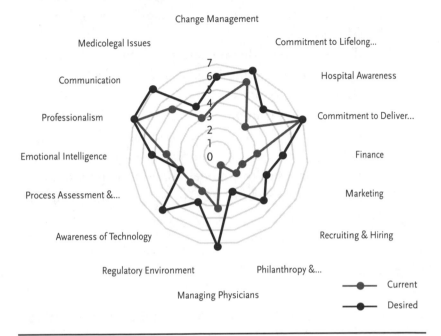

KEY TAKEAWAYS

- Understanding and managing the complexity of healthcare requires leaders with strengths that reflect administrative and EI skills and clinical and financial performance abilities.
- Effective health systems are quality centered, safe, streamlined, measured, evidence based, value driven, innovative, and equitable, and they use complementary forms of physician leadership.
- The dyad model helps mitigate the constraints of silos, improves the way clinical and business leaders work together, and optimizes the value of coordinated care.

- Effective leadership development in health systems that are also aligned with organizational goals helps sustain a pipeline of capable leaders to fill important executive and board positions.
- Studies have shown that 69 percent of physician leaders agree that doctors should be accountable for costs in addition to quality of care.
- Physician leaders gain more management and leadership skills when paired with seasoned administrators.
- Working side-by-side with business managers, who serve as active mentors or role models for aspiring physician leaders, is a valuable learning experience for practicing physicians.

REFERENCES

Angood, P., and S. Birk. 2014. "The Value of Physician Leadership." *Physician Executive* 40 (3): 6–20.

Centers for Medicare & Medicaid Services. 2016. "Medicare Accountable Care Organizations 2015 Performance Year Quality and Financial Results." Published August 25. ww.cms.gov/newsroom/fact-sheets/medicare-accountable-care-organiza tions-2015-performance-year-quality-and-financial-results.

Goodall, A. H. 2011. "Physician-Leaders and Hospital Performance: Is There an Association?" *Social Science and Medicine* 73 (4): 535–39.

Morse, G. 2010. "Health Care Needs a New Hero." *Harvard Business Review* 88 (4): 60–61.

Navigant. 2015. "69% of Physician Leaders Agree Doctors Should Be Held Accountable for Costs, in Addition to Quality of Care." Published August 3. www.navigant.com/news/healthcare/2015/physician-leadership-aapl.

Perry, J., F. Mobley, and M. Brubaker. 2017. "Most Doctors Have Little or No Management Training, and That's a Problem." *Harvard Business Review*. Published December 15. https:// hbr.org/2017/12/most-doctors-have-little-or-no-management -training-and-thats-a-problem.

Physicians Advocacy Institute. 2019. "Updated Physician Practice Acquisition Study: National and Regional Changes in Physician Employment, 2012–2018." Published February 1. www.physiciansadvocacyinstitute.org/Portals/0/assets/ docs/021919-Avalere-PAI-Physician-Employment-Trends-Study -2018-Update.pdf.

———. 2016. "Physician Practice Acquisition Study: National and Regional Employment Trends." Published September. www .physiciansadvocacyinstitute.org/Portals/0/assets/docs/Pai -Physician-employment-study.pdf.

Stoller, J. K. 2008. "Developing Physician-Leaders: Key Competencies and Available Programs." *Journal of Health Administration Education* 25 (4): 307–28.

Stoller, J. K., E. Berkowitz, and P. L. Bailin. 2007. "Physician Management and Leadership Education at the Cleveland Clinic Foundation: Program Impact and Experience over 14 Years." *Journal of Medical Practice Management* 22 (4): 237–42.

Stoller J. K., R. Coulton, and R. Kay. 2006. "A Survey of Methods of Professional Review for Physicians in Academic Medical Centers." *Journal of Medical Practice Management* 22 (3): 152–58.

Stoller, J. K., A. Goodall, and A. Baker. 2016. "Why the Best Hospitals Are Managed by Doctors." *Harvard Business Review*. Published December 27. https://hbr.org/2016/12/ why-the-best-hospitals-are-managed-by-doctors.

Index

and measures, *123–25*; guarding against suboptimization with, 125–26; origination of, 121–22; performance metrics measured with, 122–23; simplified version of, *122*; strategic value of, 126–27; transparency and, 128

Banner Health: Aetna partnership and co-branding approach with, 161

Barbati, Mike, 191

Barsoux, Jean-Louis, 289

Bates, Peter, 312

Baylor Scott & White Health's Executive Education Program (BSWEEP), 310

Becker's Hospital Review, 60, 74, 155, 184

Belasen, A. T., 296

Bhattarai, M., 181

Big data analytics, 4

Birk, Susan, 17

Bleustein, Clifford, 153

Blind spots: in doctor–patient communication, 236

Blue Cross Blue Shield of Nebraska, 138

Boards: local, advisory nature of, 6

Body language: in doctor-patient communication, 238

Bonuses: hospital value-based purchasing and, 134, *134*

Boston University Medical Campus: Advocacy Training Program, 231

"Both/and" perspective: viewing leadership tasks/responsibilities from, 309

Braddock, C. H., 229

Bradley, E. H., 181

Brand promotion and retention, 145–62; building critical mass, 146–47; convenience, 155; demand for physicians, 156–57,

158–59; excess capacity, 149–50; hospital–physician alignment, 150–53; marketing communication and co-branding, 159–61; patient wait times, 153; shortening wait times, 154–55; strategic considerations, 147–49

BSC. *See* Balanced scorecard (BSC)

BSWEEP. *See* Baylor Scott & White Health's Executive Education Program (BSWEEP)

Build: in competing values framework, *26,* 28; dyad leadership and, *30*

Bullying, 212

Bundled payments, 54, 103, 179; challenges with, 90–91; interdisciplinary structure and, 15–16; risk stratification and, 90–91

Burnout, 212; lower perceptions of patient safety culture and, 213; micromanagement and, 292; physicians and, 152; stress and, 288

Business managers: aspiring physician leaders working with, 320, 324

Butcher, Lola, 185

Byers, Jeff, 152

Capitated payment contracts: provider-owned health plans and, 137

Care coordination: team-based, 71, 75

Career development: leadership development and, 320

Care gap reports, 192

Care plans, conflicting, 178

Care teams: effective, creating, 71; physician leaders of, 306

Care transitions: improving, Partnership for Patients and, 63

CAS. *See* Complex adaptive systems (CAS)

Clever, S. L., 264
Clinical data systems: integrated health systems and, 193–94
Clinical integration (CI): adaptive culture and success of, 107; benefits of, 193–94; CI champion complementary roles and, *50*; definition of, 182; dyad leadership and, 1, 30, *30*; meeting goals for Triple Aim and, 179, 180; pillars of, 189; successful, achieving, 180–81, 184, 186; sustainable linkages between community needs and, 29; target area and clinical integration champion responsibilities, *32*
Clinical integration (CI) champion dyad role, *177*; aligning Cleveland Clinic Academy curriculum with, *322*; average ratings for, played by the dyad, 47; clinical integration target area and responsibilities of, *32*; complementary clinical integration roles and, *50*; distributed and shared roles, *35–36*; dyad evaluation survey, *42–43*; dyad leadership and, 30, *30*; dyad leadership at senior-level management and, *46*; dyads in health systems and, 30, *30*; efficiency culture type and, *108*, 109; hierarchical message orientations and, 298; personality traits and domains of action associated with, *286*; relative strengths of administrative–physician dyad and, *45*; skills and knowledge areas and, *308*
Clinical leaders: collegial orientation of, 2
Clinically integrated networks (CINs): aligning incentives and, 189–90; benefits of, 184;

components of, 184; consolidation of hospitals into, 177; Federal Trade Commission requirements met by, 182–83; physician leaders and success of, 168; technology infrastructure and, 192
Clinically vulnerable patients: shared savings and, 80
Clinical performance measures: developing, 190
Clinical preventive services, 198
Clinical programs, 190, 192
Clinical variation: measuring, 73
Closed-loop communication: soft skills and, 259
CMS. *See* Centers for Medicare & Medicaid Services (CMS)
Coaching, 311; executive, 321; sustaining leadership skills through, 320. *See also* Mentoring and mentorship
Co-branding: healthcare and hospital system, 161; marketing communication and, 159–60, 162
Collaboration: action, reflection, and, 28; clinical integration and increase in, 193; interfunctional, 178, 189, 308; interprofessional, creating culture of, 197
Collaboration, a platform for, 189–95; aligning incentives, 189–90; benefits of clinical integration, 193–94; clinical programs, 190, 192; technology infrastructure, 192
Collaboration culture type, *108*, *113*, 117; characteristics of, 111–12; diagnosing, survey methodology for, *115*; gap between actual and desired culture, *116*; patient advocate dyad role and, 109
Collaborative behavior, modeling, 220

Collaborative communication, 270, 271

Commercial insurance rate: decline in, 130

Commercial payers: price negotiations and, 136

Communication: careful, 295; closed-loop, soft skills and, 259; collaborative, 270, 271; gaps in, 229–30; open, promoting teamwork and, 212–13; paraverbal, 238; perspectives on, 296; with stakeholders, 72; through stories, 70; trust and, 18. *See also* Doctor–patient communication (DPC); Message orientation; Trust

Community-Based Care Transition program, 63–64

Community-based (or regional) populations, 68

Community health: improved, clinical integration and, 194

Community health centers: power dynamics, shifting costs, and, 136

Community hospitals, 5

Community needs: sustainable linkages between clinical integration and, 29

Community preventive services, 198

Competency development, 305–13; knowledge areas: applied management, analytics, and strategy, 307–9, *308*; mentoring and, 309, 311–12; stages of, 306–7, *307*; steps in, 309, *311*

Competing values framework (CVF): articulation of message orientations and, 26; context and roles, 30–31; definition of, 25; healthcare leadership and, *26*; interconnected axes of, 28–29; message orientation in each quadrant of, 296, *297*; uses for, 25, 26

Competition in healthcare market: benefits for consumers and, 183; hospital–physician alignment and, 152; "Pathways to Success" and, 95

Complex adaptive systems (CAS), 19–21; punctuated equilibrium and, 20; reframing challenges to integrated care with, 21; success of, 20

Complexity: ambidexterity and, 18–21

Conflict resolution, 321

Congressional Budget Office (CBO): new estimates for premium support system, 131–32

Conn, Richard, 155

Conscientiousness, 291–92; in Cross-Traits model, 285, *286*; excess of, 291, *292*, 294; in personality assessment questionnaire, *287*

Consolidation(s): pace of, in healthcare, 6, 16; physician employment trends and, 319; power dynamics, shifting costs, and, 136. *See also* Acquisitions; Mergers

Consultation dimension: in Doctor–Patient Communication Assessment, 238, *242*, *245*

Continuous improvement: dyad roles: self-assessment and, 39, 52; initiatives, balanced scorecards and, 123

Continuum of care, 5, 16, 67; dyad leaders' responsibility for, 121; integrated, 193; silos and limited coordination across, 178; Triple Aim and essential components of, 54; value-based, integrated, cooperative marketing opportunities and, 145

Convenience, 155

Convergence across healthcare fields, 4

Coordination of care, 120, 177; incentivizing, ACO model and, 93; megasystems and, 5

COPD. *See* Chronic obstructive pulmonary disease (COPD)

Cosgrove, Delos "Toby," 319

Cost control: consolidation and, 4; Triple Aim and, 53, 54

Cost shifting: power dynamics and, 136

Counseling competency: in Doctor–Patient Communication Assessment, 237, *243*; potential gaps between actual and ideal level of, *257*

Critical access hospitals, 16

Cross-training: shared team responsibility and, 211–12, 222

CrossTraits model, 285–86, *286*

CrowdMed, 62

Crowdsourcing, in healthcare, 60, 62, 64

C-suites: new positions added to, 7, 10

Cultural assessment, 112, *113*

Cultural competence: doctor–patient communication and, 239

Culture(s): "destination center" programs and, 155; diagnosing, 112; local, corporatization of, 6; of performance and competition, 109; shaping, dyad leaders and, 107; types of, *108*, 108–12, 117

Customer experience domain (or quadrant): in balanced scorecard, 122, *122*

CVF. *See* Competing values framework (CVF)

Dashboards: scorecards vs., 122

Da Vinci Surgical System, 160

Decision support systems (DSSs): RAND report and review of, 151

Defined populations, 68

Delegation: by physicians, 211, 221

Demand for physicians: FTE demand projections per 100,000 population, US, 157, *158–59*; growth in, 156–57, 162; national benchmarks for specialty groups and, 157, 162; population growth and, 157; projected physician shortage and, 157

Denver Health, 81–82

"Destination center" programs: benefits of, 155

Develop: in competing values framework, *26, 28*; dyad leadership and, *30*

Development step: in progression of learning for competency development, 309, *311*

Diabetes: CMS-HCC risk adjustment model and, 91

Diagnostic imaging systems: intraoperative, rising demand for, 146

Dignity Health: Catholic Health integrated with, 6; consolidation with Sutter Health, 136; Provider Resources, 137

Directional goals: dyad leaders and, 167

Disability compensation, patient advocates and guidance on, 226

Discharge consultation: impact on readmission rates, 181

Discrete populations: definition and examples of, 68

Diseconomies of scale, 6, 10. *See also* Economies of scale

Disproportionate Share Hospital (DSH) payments, 81, 84, 130

Doctor–patient communication (DPC), 223, 235–47; blind spots and sweet spots in, 235–36; meaningful, positive outcomes of, 228, 231; patient ratings of

Dyad patient advocate, context for, 225–32. *See also* Patient advocate dyad role

Dyad roles: aligning Cleveland Clinic Academy curriculum with, 321–22, *322*; message orientation and, 296–98; personality traits associated with, *286*, 293. *See also individual dyad roles*

Dyad roles, self-assessment, 39–52; combined strengths of the dyad across the roles, *47*; comparing relative strengths, 48–51; dyad leadership at senior-level management, *46*; gathering and representing information, 39–40; overcoming blind spots, 45–46; overlapping roles and combined strengths, 46–47

Dyads: aims in combined strength of, 23; effectiveness of, important questions about, 9; growth strategy of integrated health system and, 306; in health systems, *30*; information gathering in objective analysis of, 39–40, 44–45; synergy created by, 7–8

Dyad structure: complexity and, 318–19; critics of, 320; as a learning incubator, 320–21

Dyad value strategist, context for, 121–28. *See also* Value strategist dyad role

Eastern Maine Health System (EMHS): hospital network of, 169

Eastern Maine Medical Center (EMMC), 168–74; background, 169; establishing as a high-performing medical group, 171–73; financial metrics, 173; Five Work Streams and Medical Group

standards at, 171–72; FTI Consulting's role in creating productivity targets for, 169–71; hospitalists, clinical throughput, and length of stay, 172–73; Medical Group Oversight Committee developed at, 171; multidisciplinary rounds (MDRs) instituted at, 173; perioperative care, 172; Physician Leadership Council developed at, 171; testimonials, 173–74

Eathorne, Scott, 185

Economies of scale, 10, 109, 119; achieving, 4; hospital integration and, 17–18; mitigating factors with, 6; power dynamics, shifting costs, and, 136

Economies of scope, 120

Efficiency: increasing, balanced scorecard and, 127

Efficiency culture type, *108, 113,* 117; characteristics of, 110–11; CI champion dyad role and, *108,* 109; diagnosing, survey methodology for, *115*; gap between actual and desired culture, *116*

EHRs. *See* Electronic health records (EHRs)

EI. *See* Emotional intelligence (EI)

Electronic health record (EHR) Incentive Program: interoperability and information exchange in, 89, *90*

Electronic health records (EHRs): interoperable, enhanced use of, 95; meaningful use of, 179; templates for guiding data collection, 210

Electronic health record (EHR) system: investing in, 192, 195

Electronic medical records (EMRs): leveraging on knowledge asset dynamics through introduction of, 22

Elmore, Charles, 102
EMHS. *See* Eastern Maine Health System (EMHS)
EMMC. *See* Eastern Maine Medical Center (EMMC)
Emotional intelligence (EI), 276, 318, 321; measuring your strengths and weaknesses, *281–82*; physician leaders and, 307, 313
Emotional intelligence leaders: dyad partners as, 277–83
Emotional intelligence (EI) skills: assessing, 278–79; developing, 278, 283; diagnosing and analyzing, *280*; positive interpersonal relationships and, 278
Emotionally intelligent leaders, 277–78
Empathizing competency: in Doctor–Patient Communication Assessment, 237, *243*; potential gaps between actual and ideal level of, *252*
Empathy, 228, 232, 235, 237, 277, 279
Empathy dimension: in Doctor–Patient Communication Assessment, 238, *241, 244*
Empathy skills: current/desired, measuring, *282*; diagnosing and analyzing, *280*; leaders and emotional control through, 277
Employees: motivating, 69–70
Empowering patients: population health through, 73
EMRs. *See* Electronic medical records (EMRs)
Entrepreneurs in Residence (Cisco), 61
Epps, H. R., 229
Erickson, T. J., 220
Ethnicity in intercultural physician–patient interactions: developing sensitivity to, 239

Evans, Jenna M., 21
Event reporting, 203, 205
Evidence-based practices: engaging leaders in, 69
Excess capacity, 149–50
Executive dyads: evolving role of, 2
Exploitation, 22; complex adaptive systems and, 20; opportunities for, 23
Exploration, 22; complex adaptive systems and, 20
Extroversion, 285

Facial expressions: doctor–patient communication and, 238
Facilitating competency: in Doctor–Patient Communication Assessment, 237, *243*; potential gaps between actual and ideal level of, *256*
Falls, 59
Federal hospitals, 5
Federal poverty level (FPL): ACA's expanded Medicaid coverage and, 130
Federal Trade Commission, 139; clinically integrated networks and requirements of, 182–83
Feedback: doctor–patient communication and, 235, 246, 247; establishing safe culture for, 210; team members and, 212
Fee-for-service (FFS) payments: ACOs and, 87; fragmented, moving away from, 16
Financial incentives: hospital value-based purchasing and, 134, *134*; for provider-owned health plans, 137, 140
Financial integration, 4
Financial management: value strategist complementary roles and, *49*

Hospital Consumer Assessment
of Healthcare Providers and
Systems (HCAHPS) survey,
263–71; distinguishing factors,
266–67; doctor–patient communication and, 264, 266; goal of,
263; impact of written comments
on global outcome measures,
267–68; key percentiles for 11
publicly reported measures, 264,
265; number of patients receiving, 263, 271; perceptual gap,
268–71, *269,* 271
Hospital culture, *108*; identifying,
survey methodology for, 112,
113–15, 116
Hospital Engagement Networks
(HEN), 63
Hospital expenditures: growth in, 78
Hospital Improvement Innovation
Networks (HIINs), 63–64
Hospital–physician alignment,
150–53, 162; overarching goal of,
153; simultaneous competition
and interdependency and, 152;
technology infrastructure issues
and, 192; value creation and, 151
Hospital readmissions. *See*
Readmissions
Hospital Readmissions Reduction Program (HRRP): CMS
proposed rule and magnitude of
penalties, 82; scrutiny of, 81
Hospitals: advent of Affordable Care
Act and, 3; AHCA, negative
operating margins, and, 131;
capturing of market's healthcare
business by, 147; closure of, 4;
community, 5; consolidation
of, into clinically integrated
networks, 177; consolidation
of, into integrated healthcare
systems, 4; critical access, 16;

doctor-to-patient communication and patient ratings of, 264,
266, 271; economies of scale and
greater integration of, 17–18;
equal weighting of performance
measures/dimensions for, 79,
84; federal, 5; for-profit, 5;
full-service, 146; increases in
uncompensated care, 129; low
profitability margins and, 135,
140; nonfederal, 5; nonprofit, 5;
number of, 4–5, 5; number of
physicians employed by, 319;
performance improvement in,
22; safety net, 81–82, 83, 84; size
of, 4–6; slumping Medicare margins and, 133–35; specialty, 146;
stand-alone, decrease in, 16; state
or local government, 5; technical
assistance offered to, by QIO, 59;
traditional, supervisory structure
of, 15; VBP Program and, 79–80
Hospitals and Health Networks, 312
Hospital Survey on Patient Safety
Culture (AHRQ): composite-
level average percent positive response—2016 database
hospitals (Westat et al.), 205,
206; development of, 203, 205;
patient safety culture composites
and definitions, *204–5*
Howard, David H., 138
HRRP. *See* Hospital Readmissions
Reduction Program (HRRP)
Hudali, T., 181
Huddles, 210, 211
Human error: psychology of, 199
Humanistic approach: to leadership,
rationalistic approach used with,
29, 37
Human resources (HR) departments:
team building programs and,
220–21

Humber River Hospital: balanced scorecard dimensions/measures, 126

Huppertz, J., 267

Hybrid operating room global market value: projected increase in, 146–47

ICD-10-CM guidelines, 91

Incentives: aligning, clinically integrated networks and, 189–90; quality goals and alignment of, 4. *See also* Financial incentives

Informed decision-making: communication gaps and, 229

Injuries, 59

Innovate: in competing values framework, *26,* 28; dyad leadership and, *30*

Innovation: crowdsourced, 60, 62; culture of, 108; open, 60, 61

Innovation and learning domain (or quadrant): in balanced scorecard, 122, *122*

Innovation culture type, *108, 113,* 117; diagnosing, survey methodology for, *114;* dynamics of change and resistance in, 109; gap between actual and desired culture, *116;* innovation dyad role and, 109

Inova: Aetna partnership and cobranding approach with, 161

Inpatient Prospective Payment System, 16

Institute for Healthcare Improvement (IHI): principles for reducing wait times, 154; Triple Aim of, 53–54

Integrated approach, 25–37; context and roles in, 30–31; framework axes and, 28–29; management and leadership in, 27–28; organizing schema for, 31

Integrated health systems: dyad congruent with growth strategy of, 8

Integration: CAS framework and, 21; financial, 4; horizontal, 4; trust and, 16–18; vertical, 4, 17

Interacting competency: in Doctor–Patient Communication Assessment, 237, *243;* potential gaps between actual and ideal level of, *251*

Interaction competencies: assessment of, in DPCA, 249, *250–57*

Interdisciplinary structure: bundled payments and, 15–16

Interfunctional collaboration, 178, 189, 308

Internal business domain (or quadrant): in balanced scorecard, 122, *122*

Internal/external axis: in competing values framework, *26,* 28, 30, *30*

Internal Medicine, 80

Interoperability programs, 192

Interpersonal tasks: physician leadership development and, 306, *307*

Intuition: emotionally intelligent leaders and, 279

IT infrastructure: clinical integration and effective implementation of, 184, 186

James M. Anderson Center for Health Systems Excellence, 200

Job stress: inverse relationship between job performance and, 286, *288*

Johns Hopkins University, School of Public Health, 92

Joint Commission, The: Center for Transforming Healthcare, 198, 202; patient rights and, 225

Jones, Gareth, 278

Journal of the American Medical Association (JAMA), 16
Just culture, 199

Kaplan, Robert, 121

Labor Analytics, 170, 171
Labor expense management: at Eastern Maine Medical Center, FTI Consulting's role in, 169–70
Late arrivals policies, 154
Leaders: aspiring, traits in, 289; authentic, 280; emotionally intelligent, 277–78; engaging in evidence-based practices, 69; managers vs., 276, 277. *See also* Dyad leaders; Physician leaders
Leadership: balanced, essential importance of, 27; in collaboration culture, 111; in efficiency culture, 110; in innovation culture, 109; management and, 27–28; in performance culture, 110; safety culture and essential role of, 199, 207; situational, 293, 294, 321. *See also* Dyad leadership; Physician leadership
Leadership development: career development and, 320. *See also* Competency development
Leadership roles: changes in, 6–7; overlapping, for leading complex health systems, *31–33*
Leadership style, awareness of, 280
Learning: action learning, 320; competence approach to, 309; experiential, competency development and, 309, 313; progression of, in competency development, *311*
Learning culture, 199
Listening: active, 259; assertiveness and, 291

Listening competency: in Doctor–Patient Communication Assessment, 237, *243*; potential gaps between actual and ideal level of, *253*
Little, Kevin, 191
Living wills, patient advocates and guidance on, 226
Logos, in marketing strategies, 160
Louisiana: AHCA and negative operating margins in, 131

MACRA. *See* Medicare Access and CHIP Reauthorization Act of 2015 (MACRA)
Magnetic resonance imaging (MRI): overuse of, NCQA benchmark and, 150
Maine: AHCA and negative operating margins in, 131
Makarem, S., 266
Malpractice suits: emotional aspects of doctor–patient communication and, 228, 231
Management: bounds of, 28; leadership and, 27–28
Managers: leaders vs., 276, 277
Marketing: cooperative, 145
Marketing communication: co-branding and, 159–61
Massachusetts General Hospital: decrease in "low utility" studies at, 151
Mayo Center for Innovation, 60
Mayo Clinic, 321; Care Network, 160; Center for Innovation, review of, 60; Employee and Community Health practice, 92
McWilliams, J. Michael, 91
Meaningful use (MU), 89, 179, 192
Median operating cash-flow margins: decline in, 146

Medicaid, 136; ACA and expansion of, 82, 130; growth in spending, 77; increased payments for, 130; rate setting by, 129; underpayments, 134, 135, 140

"Medical detectives," 62

Medical errors, 54, 203

Medical groups: physician leaders of, 306

Medical schools: patient advocacy training and, 231

Medical specialties: projected shortages in, 157

Medicare, 226; CBO's examination of two federal contribution options, 132–33, *133*; growth in spending, 77; increased payments for, 129; rate setting by, 129; severity diagnosis-related group payments, 79; slumping margins for, 133–35; Trust Funds, 95; underpayments, 134, 135, 140

Medicare Access and CHIP Reauthorization Act of 2015 (MACRA), 88–89; passage of, 88; track 1+, reporting requirements, and, 96

Medicare Advantage, 132

Medicare Imaging Demonstration (MID) project: RAND Corporation report on, 151

Medicare Physician Fee Schedule, 89

Medicare rates: commercial rates and, 136

Medicare Shared Savings Program (MSSP): "Pathways to Success" proposed rule for, 95

Medicare Shared Savings Program (MSSP) ACOs: historical participation and performance, *94*; number of, 88

Medication adherence: doctor–patient communication and, 235, 258

Medication nonadherence: as public health threat, 230, 231

Megasystems: market share and, 5

Memorial Sloan Kettering (MSK) Cancer Alliance, 160

Mentoring and mentorship: developing physician leaders and, 309, 311–12, 313; effective, 311; sustaining leadership skills through, 320

Mergers, 182; among Catholic-owned hospital systems, 5–6; legal challenges and, 139; lower hospital profitability margins and, 135; waves of, 44. *See also* Acquisitions; Consolidation(s)

Merit-based Incentive Payments System (MIPS), 89, *90*

Message orientation, 295–303; appropriate messages, advantages of creating, 301–3; articulating, competing values framework and, 26; communication perspectives, 296; competing frames, recognizing in, 298, 303; current and desired, *302*; dyad roles and, 296–98; matching to different constituencies, 298, *299*; measuring, survey methodology for, *300–301*

Metzler, D. O., 229

Michigan Health & Hospital Association (MHA): partnership with Center for Transforming Healthcare, 202

Micromanagers: excess assertiveness and, 291–92

Middle managers: in collaboration culture, 112

Mintzberg, Henry, 28

MIPS. *See* Merit-based Incentive Payments System (MIPS)

Motivation skills: current/desired, measuring, *282*; diagnosing and

Per capita cost of healthcare: ACOs and, 87; reducing, 77–84

Perfectionism, 289

Performance: management centered on, 27

Performance analytics, 192

Performance culture type, *108, 113,* 117; diagnosing, survey methodology for, *114;* dynamics of change and resistance in, 110; gap between actual and desired culture, *116;* value strategist dyad role and, 109

Personality assessment: benefits of, 285, 293; questionnaire, *287*

Personality traits, 285–94; CrossTraits model, 285–86; agreeableness, 292–93; assertiveness, 290–91; conscientiousness, 291–92; dyad roles associated with, *286,* 293; openness, 288–90; stress and trait extremes, 286–88

Pharmaceutical management: improved, clinical integration and, 194

Physician leaders: aspiring, characteristics for, 8; aspiring, stages of skill building for, 306, *307,* 313; case for, 305; demand for, 310; mentoring and, 309, 311–12, 313; success of clinically integrated network and, 168; success of integrated health systems and, 316

Physician leadership: complementary forms of, 318–19, 323; skills and competencies in, *275;* value of, 17

Physician Leadership Forum, 8

Physician-led accountable care organizations (ACOs), 100–101, 103

Physician Quality Reporting System (PQRS), 89, *90*

Physicians: burnout and, 152; clinical integration and expectations/incentives for, 184, 186; communication gaps and, 229; delegation and, 211, 221; demand for, 156–57, *158–59,* 162; employed by health systems, 5; empowering, autonomy and discretion in, 180–81; expanded role for, in hospital leadership, 3; heroic lone healer myth and, 318; hospital-employed, 319; interpersonal communication skills of, 235, 246; patient wait times and, 153; projected shortage of, 157; as ultimate patient advocates, 223; virtual visits with, 159. *See also* Doctor–patient communication (DPC); Hospital–physician alignment; Primary care physicians

Physicians Advocacy Institute (PAI), 5, 319

Physician services expenditures: growth in, 78

POHPs. *See* Provider-owned health plans (POHPs)

Population growth: physician demand and, 157, 162

Population health, 67–75, 77; benefits of, 67; challenges with, 67; dyad leadership and, 30, *30;* health innovator complementary roles and, *48;* improving, Triple Aim and, 53, 54; target area and health innovator responsibilities, *31;* through empowering patients, 73; types of, 68

Population health (health innovator): distributed and shared roles, *33;* dyad evaluation survey, *40–41*

RAND Corporation report: on Medicare Imaging Demonstration (MID) project, 151

Rate limiting: managing, 154

Rationalistic approach: humanistic approach to leadership used with, 29, 37

Readmissions: reducing, 16, 181–82, 186

Reason, James: on elements of safety culture, 199

Redundancy: reducing or eliminating, 4

Reflection: management and, 28

Rege, Alyssa, 184

Regional hubs: consolidated services in, 5

Regional populations: definition of, 68

Reimbursement: encounter-based, shift away from, 177; evolving pay structures and, 318; factors related to transitions in, 119; low hospital profitability margins and, 135; power dynamics, cost shifting, and, 136; provider-owned insurers and, 138. See also Bundled payments; Fee-for-service payments

Relational goals: dyad leaders and, 167

Relational message orientation, 296–97, 297; current and desired profile, 302; matching to different constituencies, 299

Reliability culture. See Safety and reliability culture

Reporting culture, 199

Resistance: in innovation culture, 109; in performance culture, 110

Respectful patient treatment, 226, 228, 232

Respecting competency: in Doctor–Patient Communication Assessment, 237, 243; potential

gaps between actual and ideal level of, 250

Risk-based cost model: developing, 190, 194

Risk management, 54

Risk stratification, 54; aims of, 92; bundled payments and, 90–91

Robinson, R., 181

Rogers, P. S., 296

Role clarity, understanding, 221

Rounding: in high-reliability organizations, 200

Rural hospitals: in Medicaid expansion and nonexpansion states, 131

Safety and reliability culture: fitting into, 197–207; leadership's essential role in, 199, 207; promoting, 198. See also Patient safety

Safety net hospitals, 81–82, 84; HRRP and disproportionate penalties for, 83

Same-day appointments, 156

Sanborn, Beth Jones, 135

Sanford, Deborah, 174

Saunders, Ninfa, 184

Scale: in competing values framework, 26, 28; dyad leadership and, 30

Scheduling errors: reducing, 154

Schwartz, Aaron L., 91

Scorecards: dashboards vs., 122. See also Balanced scorecard (BSC)

Scripted communication style, 243

Secure messaging, 192

Self-assessments: gathering and representing information in, 39–40, 44–45; uses for, 39

Self-awareness skills, 277, 318; current/desired, measuring, 281; developing, 307; diagnosing and analyzing, 280; leaders, emotional control, and, 277; personality assessment and, 285

Sunnybrook Health Sciences Centre: strategic mapping example, 126
Surgical procedures: coordinated roles and responsibilities for, 213
Surgical site infections, 59
Sustainable growth rate (SGR), 89
Sutter Health: consolidation with Dignity Health, 136
Sweet spots: in doctor–patient communication, 236
Synergy as strategy, 7–8, 10

Tactical dashboards: balanced scorecards vs., 126
Talent pipeline, building, 315, 317
Task ambiguity, understanding, 221
Team-based care coordination, 71, 75
Team leadership: evolution of, through transition phases, 219
Teamwork, 178; assessment and development of, 209–22; cross-training and shared responsibility in, 211–12, 222; decision-making process and, 209; gaining buy-in and, 220–21; mapping, 219; open communication and, 212–13; promoting, 307
Teamwork survey: aggregate ratings of team members across eight composites of, 217, 218, 219, 220; behavioral characteristics of effective teamwork, 213, 214; conducting, 217; methodology, 215–17
Technical tasks: physician leadership development and, 306, 307
Technology: including in marketing strategies, 160; infrastructure, clinically integrated networks and, 192
Testing, eliminating redundant, 190
Thackway McCord, 161

THN. *See* Together Health Network (THN), Michigan
360-degree feedback, 321
Toegel, Ginka, 289
Together Health Network (THN), Michigan: as "super CIN," 185
Tone of voice: doctor–patient communication and, 238
Tongue, J. R., 229
Total performance score (TPS), 79
Traditional approaches: to leadership development, 317
Transactional perspective: communication from, 296, 303
Transformational mentors, 311
Transformational message orientation, 297, 298; current and desired profile, 302; matching to different constituencies, 299
Transformational perspective: communication from, 296, 303
Transformations in healthcare field, 3–4
Transition management, training in, 308
Transition of care (TOC) clinic attendance: negative predication for readmission and, 181
Transparency: balanced scorecard and, 128; culture of safety and reliability and, 198; "destination center" programs and, 155; promoting a safety culture and, 213
Transparency Market Research, 146
Trinity Health, 185
Triple Aim (IHI), 53, 68, 77; ACOs and pursuit of, 87; articulation of goals, 53; central focus of, 54; clinical integration and support for, 179, 180; clinically integrated networks and goals of, 178; requirements for achieving goals of, 57

Trish, Erin E., 138

Trust: communication and, 18; culture of safety and reliability and, 198; doctor–patient communication and, 223, 235, 239, 246; Fellows of the American College of Surgeons on, 227; integration and, 16–18; of internal/external stakeholders, earning, 27; mutual, in closed-loop communication, 259; respectful patient treatment and, 228; teamwork and, 209

Tsasis, Peter, 21

Turnover rates: for CEOs, 7, 315

Two-sided risk models, transition to, 95

Uncompensated care: American Health Care Act and cost increases for, 131; hospital increases in, 129

Undercommunicating, 295

Uninsured population: ACA, Medicaid expansion, and, 130; safety net hospitals and, 81

United States: medication nonadherence in, 230; number of hospitals in, 4–5, 5; physician burnout in, 152

Unity Health, 160

University Hospitals: Aetna partnership and co-branding approach with, 161

University of Michigan Health System, 185

Update step: in progression of learning for competency development, 309, 311

US Department of Health and Human Services (HHS), 79; Office of Inspector General, 88;

Partnership for Patients initiative, 59

US Department of Justice, 183

Validating competency: in Doctor–Patient Communication Assessment, 237, 243; potential gaps between actual and ideal level of, 254

Value: creating through process mapping, 191; promoting, balanced scorecard and, 127

Value-based care arrangements: provider-owned health plans and, 137

Value-based contracting: clinical integration and, 189

Value-based payment methods: shift to, 178

Value Based Payment Modifier (VBM), 89, 90

Value-based purchasing (VBP), 79–80, 84

Value strategist: domain of operation, dyad leadership and, 168; primary objective of, in healthcare organizations, 120

Value strategist dyad role, 119; aligning Cleveland Clinic Academy curriculum with, 322; average ratings for, played by the dyad, 47; complementary financial management roles and, 49; dyad leadership at senior-level management and, 46; dyads in health systems and, 30, 30; financial performance target area and responsibilities of, 32; handling of key internal/external interfaces and, 168, 174; performance culture and, 109; personality traits and domains of action associated

About the Author

Alan Belasen, PhD, is an experienced leadership development coach; consultant; and trainer in business, nonprofit, and government organizations in the United States and abroad. He led the design and implementation of master's in business administration programs in management, global leadership, and healthcare leadership at the State University of New York (SUNY) Empire State College, and he chaired all three for many years. Dr. Belasen has published extensively on topics such as executive education, self-managed teams, human resources competencies, motivation, women's leadership, communication innovation, corruption in business, trusted leadership, middle management, corporate communication, reputation management, and healthcare communication. His articles have appeared in the *Journal of Health Organization and Management, Economic Modelling, Academy of Management Proceedings, Journal of Health Administration and Education*, and *Journal of Management Development*. His most recent books are *Women in Management: A Framework for Sustainable Work–Life Integration* (Routledge, 2017) and *Mastering Leadership: A Vital Resource for Health Care Organizations* (Jones & Bartlett, 2015). Dr. Belasen is a recipient of the IACBE John L. Green Award for Excellence in Business Education and the SUNY Chancellor's Award for Scholarship and Creative Activities.